teach ®
yourself

aromatherapy

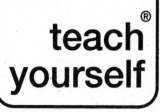

teach yourself®

aromatherpy
denise whichello brown,
B.Sc., Cert. Ed., D.O.,
M. A.O., M.I.F.P.A., M.I.F.R.

For over 60 years, more than
40 million people have learnt over
750 subjects the **teach yourself**
way, with impressive results.

be where you want to be
with **teach yourself**

For UK order enquiries: please contact Bookpoint Ltd, 130 Milton Park, Abingdon, Oxon OX14 4SB. Telephone: +44 (0) 1235 827720. Fax: +44 (0) 1235 400454. Lines are open 09.00–18.00, Monday to Saturday, with a 24-hour message answering service. Details about our titles and how to order are available at www.teachyourself.co.uk

For USA order enquiries: please contact McGraw-Hill Customer Services, PO Box 545, Blacklick, OH 43004-0545, USA. Telephone: 1-800-722-4726. Fax: 1-614-755-5645.

For Canada order enquiries: please contact McGraw-Hill Ryerson Ltd, 300 Water St, Whitby, Ontario L1N 9B6, Canada. Telephone: 905 430 5000. Fax: 905 430 5020.

Long renowned as the authoritative source for self-guided learning – with more than 40 million copies sold worldwide – the **teach yourself** series includes over 300 titles in the fields of languages, crafts, hobbies, business, computing and education.

British Library Cataloguing in Publication Data: a catalogue record for this title is available from the British Library.

Library of Congress Catalog Card Number: on file.

First published in UK 1996 by Hodder Education, 338 Euston Road, London, NW1 3BH.

First published in US 1996 by Contemporary Books, a Division of the McGraw-Hill Companies, 1 Prudential Plaza, 130 East Randolph Street, Chicago, IL 60601 USA.

This edition published 2003.

The **teach yourself** name is a registered trade mark of Hodder Headline.

Typeset by Transet Limited, Coventry, England.
Printed in Great Britain for Hodder Education, a division of Hodder Headline, 338 Euston Road, London NW1 3BH, by Cox & Wyman Ltd, Reading, Berkshire.

Hodder Headline's policy is to use papers that are natural, renewable and recyclable products and made from wood grown in sustainable forests. The logging and manufacturing processes are expected to conform to the environmental regulations of the country of origin.

Impression number   7 6 5 4
Year   2009 2008 2007 2006 2005

v

contents

In loving memory of my dear friend Peter Grant, a true believer in the art of aromatherapy, who passed away shortly before the completion of this book.

introduction

Aromatherapy has become one of the fastest growing natural healing arts in this country. It is rapidly gaining respect from orthodox medical practitioners, and qualified clinical aromatherapists who now work not only from their own private practices but also in hospitals, hospices and surgeries.

The art of aromatherapy uses pure essential oils which are extracted from various parts of plants and trees. These natural, aromatic, liquid substances, often considered to be the 'life force' or 'soul' of plants, are endowed with a whole host of therapeutic properties. They are remarkably versatile and may be used in various ways. This book aims to show you how to use essential oils *safely* and effectively on your friends and family without creating harmful side effects, unlike many chemical drugs. The information contained within these pages will also be invaluable to the student or practising aromatherapist.

Aromatherapy is a holistic therapy which can be used to promote physical, mental and spiritual health equilibrium. It forms part of a holistic healing régime which involves searching for the root causes of an illness rather than its symptoms and awakening the body's innate ability to heal itself, leading to a state of balance. Aromatherapy involves far more than the application of essential oils. To achieve 'whole healing', factors such as diet and lifestyle must *always* be considered.

A great deal of this book is devoted to the 'wholistic' treatment of various conditions. I have indicated not only which essential oils should be selected on a physical, emotional and spiritual level but also which Bach Flower Remedies may be appropriate to enable us to treat the person rather than the disease. These remedies, I believe, are an invaluable accompaniment to essential oils. They aim to balance our negative states of mind, such as worry and fear, which are so depleting to our immune systems and ultimately can lead to serious disease. I have also included dietary advice for each condition which is vital if true healing is to take place. Where appropriate I have suggested other courses of action which can enhance and support the aromatherapy treatment.

Since I have stepped into the world of essential oils, my life has been completely transformed. I do hope that you will allow aromatherapy to become part of your daily life and that this book will encourage you to learn more about these fascinating, healing, essential oils which can help you to achieve balance of mind, body and spirit.

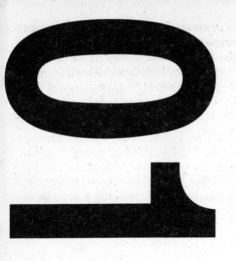

01

the history of aromatherapy

In this chapter you will learn:
- the history of aromatherapy.

Plants have been employed for medicinal purposes since the dawn of mankind. Primitive people relied very much on their instincts to keep them alive. By following their sense of smell and by drawing on their experiences they were able to acquire knowledge of how certain plants had the capacity to heal and cure ailments and diseases. When animals are sick, they instinctively search for plants which can heal and relieve their symptoms.

Early civilizations

In the caves of Lascaux in the Dordogne region of France there are cave paintings which depict the use of plants for healing and medicinal purposes. Archaeologists estimate that these paintings date back as far as 18000 BC.

A terracotta 'still' which experts believe to be 5000 years old is housed in the Taxila Museum in Pakistan. This still would have been employed for making aromatic waters and even perhaps for the production of essential oils. It is believed to have belonged to the ancient Indus or Arab civilisations. This is a curious phenomenon since distillation was thought to have been 'invented' only 1000 years ago. There is no other evidence of the use of distillation from 5000 to 1000 BC. Therefore 5000 years ago ancient civilisations must have been far more advanced than was previously thought.

Egypt

I believe that aromatherapy was born in ancient Egypt, and plant medicine dates back to at least 3000 BC. There is much evidence to suggest that aromatics formed a part of Egyptian daily life. Around 3000 BC the oldest known pyramid in Egypt, the 'Step Pyramid', was built by King Zoser at Saqqara. His chief architect was the genius Imhotep who was a renowned physician as well as an astronomer and scribe. Imhotep did a great deal to advance medical knowledge at this time and he is sometimes referred to as the 'grandfather of aromatherapy'.

The Papyrus of Ebers (1550 BC), one of the few surviving medical papyri, reveals the widespread and frequent use of aromatics in Egyptian medicine. From the papyrus it is apparent that aromatics were used both externally and internally to combat health problems. Egyptian priests prescribed medicinal wines for all sorts of conditions. Inhalations were taken for respiratory problems. Sitz baths and douches were recommended for gynaecological disorders. Gargles were employed for problems with the mouth and gums, and ointments were prepared for diseases of the skin.

The ordinary Egyptians used aromatics in their cooking for health purposes. Garlic, for instance, was highly prized for its ability to ward off disease and to prevent the outbreak of epidemics. Other herbs and spices used include aniseed, caraway, mint, marjoram and parsley.

The Egyptian perfumers were highly skilled and they formulated the famous 'Kyphi' – a favourite perfume and incense. It was a blend of sixteen aromatics. The exact ingredients of Kyphi are unknown but it is thought to have contained calamus, cinnamon, frankincense, henna, juniper and myrrh, amongst others. It was a popular item in the Egyptian home and was not only employed as a perfume and burnt as an incense but also presented as a medicine. Kyphi was inhaled during meditations to heighten spiritual awareness. Its ingredients encouraged new levels of consiousness. Frankincense was also used to increase spiritual and psychic awareness. It is fascinating that when the tomb of Tutankhamun, who ruled from 1361–52 BC, was opened in 1922 one of the sealed flasks contained an ungent which still had an aroma – despite the fact it was over 3300 years old. Frankincense was one of the aromatics contained in it.

The Egyptians were well aware of the ability of the aromas to affect the emotions. Each Pharaoh was lucky enough to have a number of different perfumes blended for him. Perfumes were formulated to uplift the spirits, dispel nervousness, encourage love, bring tranquillity and induce aggression for the purposes of war.

Perfumes and religion were closely connected. The Egyptians adorned their gods with scented oils; gods and goddesses had fragrances dedicated to them and the statues were sometimes anointed. For instance, myrrh was dedicated to the moon and frankincense to the sun-god, Ra. Aromatics were burnt during religious ceremonies as offerings to the deities. (The Latin *per fumum* means 'through smoke'.)

Wealthy Egyptian women would indulge themselves in an aromatherapy massage after a bath. The slave girls would apply the oils which rejuvenated and perfumed the skin. Cedarwood oil was a particular favourite. Egyptian women even knew about contraception. Aromatic mixtures were blended together and placed in the vagina to act as spermicides.

The Egyptians strongly believed in reincarnation and the afterlife, and when we think of Egyptians we always equate them with the process of mummification. They went to tremendous lengths in their embalming procedures and they really were experts. Many of the major organs were removed, including the brain which was hooked out through the nostrils and the abdominal viscera were also taken out. Myrrh, cassia, galbanum and other aromatic substances were employed to fill up the cavities. The blood was drained out and then the body was bathed in natron (a sodium carbonate solution). The body was left for approximately seventy days and then wrapped in bandages which had been soaked with various aromatics including cedarwood oil. Each embalmer would have his own particular recipe. The formulations were remarkably effective at preserving the human flesh and even now, after thousands of years, mummies have been discovered in a wonderful state of preservation. These elaborate procedures, of course, were employed only for the embalming of high priests and pharaohs.

The Nile Valley became known as the 'Cradle of Medicine'. Medicinal plants such as cedarwood, cinnamon, frankincense and myrrh were transported to this area to grow. When the Jews began their exodus in about 1240 BC from Egypt to Israel they departed with much knowledge and many precious gums and oils. In the Old and New Testament of the Bible there are numerous references to oils – calamus, cassia, cinnamon, hyssop and olive amongst them! Of course, frankincense and myrrh were offered to Jesus Christ at his birth.

China

Aromatic herbs and massage were used in China long before the birth of Christ. Along the Yellow River 5000 years ago the Chinese were using mugwort leaves and calamus roots for hygiene purposes. Emperor Shen Nung's medical text *Herbal* dates back to about 2700 BC and it contains details on 365 plants. Emperor Huang Ti is credited with *The Yellow Emperor's Classic of Internal Medicine* (2650 BC). In this work aromatic medicines and massage are referred to on several occasions. This book also forms much of the basis for acupuncture.

India

In India plants and plant extracts were being employed from at least 3000 BC. The oldest form of Indian medicine is known as 'Ayurvedic' and uses many different massage techniques, pressure points and also essential oils. One of the oldest known Indian books on plants called *Vedas* mentions basil, cinnamon, coriander, ginger, myrrh and sandalwood.

The Greeks

The ancient Greeks played a very important part in aromatic medicine, developing the knowledge acquired from the Egyptians.

The most renowned Greek is, of course, Hippocrates (460–370 BC) who became known as the 'Father of Medicine'. He adopted a holistic approach and advocated daily aromatic baths and massage. He wrote in his *Aphorisms* that 'aromatic baths are useful in the treatment of female disorders'.

Asclepiades (200 BC), a Greek physician, believed in gentle therapies such as bathing, massage, music, perfume and wine. He was opposed to the use of purgatives and emetics which were so popular at that time. Theophrastus, the famous Greek botanist, advocated the use of perfumes, plasters and poultices for medicinal purposes. He had noticed that oils which are applied externally can affect the internal organs. Another famous Greek was Megallus who formulated a successful preparation containing cassia, cinnamon and myrrh known as 'Megaleion', renowned throughout Greece.

The Romans

Pedacius Dioscorides of Anazarba wrote a five-volume book known as *De Materia Medica* in the first century AD. One of the volumes is full of information regarding the uses of plants and aromatics. Cypress, juniper, marjoram and myrrh are mentioned among the 500 plants described in this study. He mentions Kyphi claiming that it is calming and helps to relieve asthma attacks. Other formulae include 'Amarakinon' to treat haemorrhoids and menstrual difficulties, 'Susinon' to treat fluid retention and 'Nardinon muron' for coughs and colds. A great deal of our present knowledge of medicinal herbs comes from Dioscorides.

The Romans adored perfumes and aromatic oils and used them for massage and scenting their hair and clothing. In Rome the *hetairi* or prostitutes used scent lavishly. Galen, the physician to the gladiators, prepared ointments and he also produced a 'cold cream'.

As the Roman soldiers marched into battle they carried myrrh with them to heal their wounds. Their knowledge of the healing properties of plants spread throughout their growing Empire. Wherever they went they collected and planted seeds. In Britain, for instance, herbs such as parsley, sage, fennel, rosemary and thyme were planted.

Avicenna

Born in Persia, the physician and scholar Avicenna (AD 980–1037), is credited with the invention of distillation. There was already a crude type of distillation in operation but Avicenna refined it by extending the length of the cooling pipe and forming it into a coil. This enabled the condensation of steam and vaporised essence to be far more efficient. Rose water made from *rosa centifolia* became popular. The Persians exported it to China, Europe and India and it was used for medicinal and culinary purposes. Perfumes were formulated using roses, lilies, narcissi and violets.

Avicenna wrote almost 100 books throughout his life. His most renowned work is the *Canon of Medicine*. This book was used as a standard reference text by many medical schools for 500 years up until the middle of the sixteenth century. He mentions many essential oils including chamomile, cinnamon, dill and peppermint.

The Crusaders, during the Holy Wars, brought back knowledge of herbal medicines and perfumes, handed down from the Romans.

The Middle Ages

Religious orders cultivated their own aromatic plants – in the twelfth century the German Abbess, Hildegarde, was well known for growing lavender.

In the Middle Ages lavender and other herbs made up into bouquets were used as protection against plagues. Frankincense and pine were burned in the streets in the fourteenth century. Basil, chamomile, lavender, melissa and thyme were strewn on the ground and chamomile lawns became popular. Perfumes were used widely in England as people hardly ever washed themselves, so the perfumes masked unpleasant natural body odours.

During the sixteenth century many books were written on distillation, many of them in German. Alchemy – the practice of trying to transform base metal into gold, was widespread. In 1576, the Swiss physician and alchemist Paracelsus wrote the *Great Surgery Book*. He claimed that the role of alchemy was not to turn base metals into gold but instead to develop medicines, especially medicines from plants.

In 1597 the German Braunschweig published his book called *Neue Vollkommen Distillierbuch* containing references to twenty-five essential oils.

Throughout the Renaissance period essential oils were widely used and botany was part of the study of medicine.

The seventeenth, eighteenth and nineteenth centuries

Many English herbalists emerged during the seventeenth century – the most renowned herbalists include John Parkinson, John Gerarde and Nicholas Culpepper. In 1653 Culpepper wrote his famous *Complete Herbal*. The plague wreaked havoc once more and aromatic herbs were popular. The perfumers enjoyed an immunity to the plague because they were surrounded by essential oils. Essential oils were being used in mainstream medicine for a host of internal and external diseases.

During the eighteenth century practically all herbalists and some doctors were using essential oils. Potions were mixed up in apothecaries – each had its own still.

Scientists of the nineteenth century identified some of the chemical constituents of oils and gave them names such as 'geraniol' and 'citronellol'. Unfortunately this led to the development of synthetic copies of the main constituents of the oils. The use of herbs and essential oils declined greatly as the drug companies started to flourish. Synthetic drugs, sadly, can produce numerous side effects and can be toxic and harmful.

The twentieth century

The birth of modern aromatherapy can be attributed to the French chemist René Maurice Gattefossé. It was Gattefossé who coined the word 'aromatherapy' in 1937 with the publication of his book *Aromathérapie*. It is said that after burning his hand in an experiment, he plunged it into the nearest liquid which happened to contain lavender oil. He used essential oils on the wounds of soldiers who were injured during the First World War.

Other chemists were also investigating the use of essential oils. In Australia, Penfold and others were researching the benefits of tea tree oil. In Italy, doctors Giovanni Gatti and Renato Cayola discovered the psychotherapeutic effects of essential oils – such as jasmine and lemon.

French doctor Jean Valnet, an army surgeon who had been influenced by the work of Gattefossé, made an enormous impact on the aromatherapy world with the publication of his book *Aromathérapie* in 1964. His book is regarded by many as the aromatherapist's bible. He had used essential oils for treating war wounds and after the war he continued to use essential oils. He taught other members of the medical profession about the therapeutic effects of essential oils. In France some doctors study aromatherapy and prescribe essential oils.

Madame Marguerite Maury (1895–1964) introduced aromatherapy into Britain in the late 1950s. She applied the essential oils, diluted in a carrier oil, using massage techniques. She taught her techniques to beauty therapists and wrote a book *The Secret of Life and Youth* which is concerned with rejuvenation.

Nowadays aromatherapy is becoming an increasingly popular therapy for a wide range of ailments. It is practised by professional qualified clinical aromatherapists in hospitals, clinics, hospices and surgeries. The demand for aromatherapy is growing rapidly.

02

extracting the oils

In this chapter you will learn:
- the main methods of extracting essential oils.

There are several methods of obtaining aromatic substances from plant material, most of which I have described below. But strictly speaking, essential oils are only those obtained by distillation or expression.

Distillation

Distillation is the most widely used and the most economical method of extracting essential oils. Many historians attribute the discovery of distillation to Avicenna, the Persian physician and scholar (see Chapter 01) although possibly the Egyptians were aware of the primitive process. There is a great deal of skill involved in the process of distillation if the precious essential oil is not to be lost or changed in its composition. Some plants are distilled immediately after harvesting, whereas others may be left for a few days or even dried prior to extraction.

In distillation, the plant material is heated, either by placing it in water which is brought to the boil or by passing steam through it. The heat and steam cause the cell structure of the plant material to burst and break down, thus freeing the essential oils. The essential oil molecules and steam are carried along a pipe and channelled through a cooling tank, where they return to liquid form and are collected in a vat. The emerging liquid is a mixture of oil and water, and since essential oils are not water soluble they can be easily separated from the water and siphoned off. Essential oils which are lighter than water will float on the surface, whereas heavier oils such as clove will sink.

The water travelling around the distillation plant becomes impregnated with aroma and is recycled, and may be used as perfumed water such as lavender water or rose water.

During the process of distillation only the extremely small volatile molecules are able to evaporate. Essential oils which contain a high proportion of the smallest (most volatile) of these molecules are referred to as 'top notes'. Those which are composed mostly of the heaviest (least volatile) molecules are known as 'base notes'. Essential oils which are in between are called 'middle notes'.

Top note oils are the most volatile – the aroma disappears within twenty-four hours. Examples are basil, grapefruit, lemon, lime and eucalyptus. They tend to be stimulating and uplifting.

Middle note oils have an aroma which lasts for two to three days. Examples are chamomile, geranium and lavender. They are generally balancing and primarily affect the general metabolism and the systems of the body such as digestion and menstruation.

Base note oils are the least volatile – the aroma will last at least one week. Examples are frankincense, myrrh, neroli, patchouli and vetivert. They have a relaxing and sedative quality.

The first distillation is usually the best quality. If essential oils are redistilled this process is known as 'rectification'. The second and subsequent distillations will produce a cheaper oil unsuitable for aromatherapy.

Expression

This method is reserved exclusively for members of the citrus family such as bergamot, grapefruit, lemon, lime, mandarin and orange. The essence yielded is found in small sacs which are located under the surface of the rind. This process was originally carried out using simple hand pressure. The citrus essence was squeezed from the rinds and then collected in a sponge which, once saturated, was squeezed into a bucket. Why not try hand pressing the rind of a citrus fruit yourself? You can have your own hand expression plant in your kitchen!

Due to the labour costs involved the majority of citrus oil is now expressed using mechanical presses. A great deal of essential oil of orange is produced in the United States in fruit-juice factories. However, this is not the best oil to use as the crops are treated with pesticides and chemical fertilisers which contaminate the essence. Citrus oils for therapeutic aromatherapy use are best obtained from organically or naturally grown fruit.

Unfortunately some citrus oil factories distil the peel after expression in order to release more oil. Obviously this essential oil is of an inferior quality but it is often added to the expressed essential oil to increase the quantity and thus make more profit.

Solvent extraction

The process of solvent extraction does not yield essential oils. This method is employed for flowers, gums and resins and it produces 'absolutes' and 'resinoids'. The technique is used for higher yield or to extract oils that cannot be obtained by any other process. Jasmine, for example, is adversely affected by hot water and steam.

Absolutes

To yield an absolute the aromatic plant material (flowers, leaves, etc.) is extracted by hydrocarbon solvents such as benzene or hexane. The plant material is covered with the solvent and slowly heated to dissolve the aromatic molecules. The solvent extracts the odour and then the solvent is filtered off to produce a 'concrete'. A concrete is a solid, wax-like substance containing about 50 per cent wax and 50 per cent volatile oil such as jasmine.

To obtain the absolute the concrete is mixed with pure alcohol to dissolve out the aromatic molecules, and then chilled. This mixture is filtered to eliminate waste products and to separate out insoluble waxes. The alcohol is evaporated off gently under vacuum. The thick, viscous, coloured liquid known as the absolute is left behind.

This method is widely used for rose, jasmine and neroli. A trace of the solvent, however, will always remain. Therefore an absolute can never be as pure as an essential oil which has been extracted via the process of distillation. Absolutes are sometimes adulterated due to their high price. Take care to always buy from a reputable supplier.

Resinoids

Solvent extraction can also be used for gums and resins to produce resinoids. Resins are the solid/semi-solid substances which exude naturally from a tree or plant that has been damaged. Commercially, resins are obtained by cutting into the bark or stem, and the gum-like substance hardens once it is exposed to the air.

The natural resinous material is extracted with a hydrocarbon solvent such as petroleum ether, hexane or alcohol. These solvents are then filtered off and subsequently removed by distillation. A resinoid remains where a hydrocarbon solvent has been used (e.g. benzoin resinoid). If an alcohol solvent has been used then an absolute resin is produced (e.g. frankincense and myrrh resin absolutes may be extracted from the crude oleo resin gum – both, however, may be extracted by steam distillation to produce an essential oil).

Resinoids are often employed by the perfume manufacturers as fixatives to prolong the aroma of a fragrance (as are concretes).

Enfleurage

The process of enfleurage also yields an absolute, although this method is virtually obsolete nowadays. It is very time consuming and labour intensive and, therefore, highly expensive. Formerly this was the main method of extraction for delicate flowers such as jasmine which continue to produce perfume even after they have been picked. It involves the use of purified odourless cold fat which is spread over sheets of glass mounted in large rectangular wooden frames. Flowers are strewn upon this layer of fat which absorbs the essential oil. After approximately a day the flowers are removed to be replaced by fresh flowers. This process is repeated many times – even beyond two months – until the fat is saturated. This fragrance saturated fat is known as a 'pomade'. The pomade is washed in alcohol and then treated. The alcohol evaporates first and the pure absolute is produced.

Carbon dioxide extraction

This relatively new method was introduced only in the 1980s. The price is high because the equipment used is expensive. The process has been designed for the perfume industry. Oils which are extracted utilising carbon dioxide are supposed to be superior, pure and very close to the natural essential oil as it exists in the plant – and they are completely free of residues of carbon dioxide.

The prices are too high at the moment to be of value to the aromatherapist. However, as the costs are reduced and production increases they may become available. Research would be necessary to evaluate their therapeutic benefits since the composition of the essential oil is different.

Hydrodiffusion/percolation

Hydrodiffusion or percolation is the most modern method of extraction. This process is faster than distillation, and the equipment is much more simple than that used for carbon dioxide extraction. Steam spray is passed through the plant material (which is suspended on a grid) from above. The emerging liquid composed of oil and condensed steam is then cooled. The result is a mixture of essential oil and water (as in the distillation process) which can be easily separated. Although this method is promising, research is necessary to evaluate the place of these oils in aromatherapy.

Maceration

For this process plants are placed into a vat of warm vegetable oil which causes the plant cells to rupture, causing the absorption of the essential oils. The vat is then agitated for several days. The resulting oil is filtered and bottled, and is ready for use as a massage medium. Examples of macerated oils are calendula, carrot and hypericum.

Why not try to make your own macerated oils at home? Half fill a glass jar with your chosen plant material (e.g. lemon balm). Add your warm, good quality vegetable oil to fill up the jar. It is an excellent idea to add 10 per cent of wheatgerm oil to preserve your mixture. Screw the top on the jar and store it in a warm place for a week or so; remember to shake the jar daily. Finally filter off the plant material, rebottle and label.

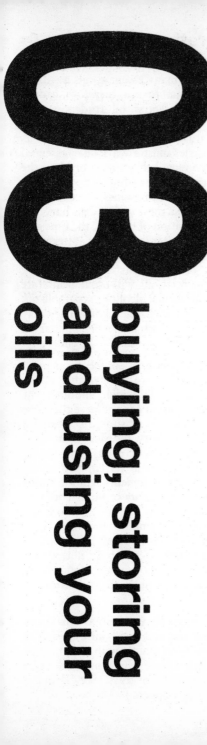

03

buying, storing and using your oils

In this chapter you will learn:
- how to recognize high quality pure essential oils
- how to look after your oils
- ways of using essential oils.

Quality and adulteration

It is vital to use only high-quality pure essential oils for optimum results. It is most unfortunate that many essential oils available on the market today are of poor quality and, therefore, cannot help alleviate health problems. Essential oil traders supply mostly to the perfume and food industries who are more concerned with the fragrance or flavour of an oil rather than its therapeutic effects. These industries must always have essential oils with the same chemical formulae if they are to produce the same aroma and taste consistently, so they find it necessary to 'adulterate' oils to replicate aromas and flavours. Price is also a major consideration. Factors such as the weather, bad harvests, the variety of the plant, the composition of the soil, the time and the method of cultivation and extraction can affect the composition of essential oils greatly and this creates difficulties for the perfume and the food industries who seek standardisation. Suppliers of essential oils will often adulterate their oils by adding synthetic ingredients, alcohols, vegetable oil, cheap chemical constituents or low-cost essential oils. They may even substitute an entire essential oil with a cheaper, similar oil for commercial gain (e.g. lavendin may be sold as lavender).

Essential oils used in aromatherapy must, of course, be as pure, natural and 'whole' as possible if they are to have the desired therapeutic effects. Synthetic materials which simulate the aroma and appearance of an essential oil cannot have the same therapeutic properties as an essential oil and should *not* be used in therapy. Synthetic chemicals also carry the risk of harmful and unpleasant side effects, as do synthetic drugs. It is totally impossible to duplicate an essential oil in its entirety in the laboratory. Vital constituents and trace elements will inevitably be missing. It is the *total* of the components of an essential oil working together which produces a healing effect. If oils are referred to as 'nature identical' this implies that the oil is synthetic and produced in the laboratory and is, therefore, unsuitable for aromatherapy. Synthetic oils also do not possess the 'vital force' or 'life force' of essential oils which comes from living plants. Chemicals also do not contain the 'vibration' of natural living plants.

Since most aromatherapy suppliers buy essential oils from importers who supply the perfume and food industries it is important to seek a supplier who deals mainly with essential oils intended only for therapeutic use. I have found over the years that purchasing essential oils is a matter of trust. (See 'Taking it Further' for information regarding suppliers.)

Care and storage

Essential oils are extremely precious and should be treated with respect – they can also be very expensive. They are damaged by ultraviolet light and deteriorate more rapidly at the blue end of the spectrum than the red. Therefore, essential oils should be stored in amber-coloured bottles (if you do keep your essential oils in blue bottles then they should be kept in the dark – this is less important if your bottles are brown). Never decant the oils into clear glass or plastic bottles. They should never be placed in direct sunlight, so avoid sunny windowsills or shelves on radiators – no matter how attractive the bottles look! Essential oils do not like extremes of temperatures. They are highly volatile which means that they evaporate rapidly. Always replace the caps immediately and ensure that the tops are tightly closed when the oils are not in use.

Pure essential oils will last for approximately three years from the bottling date. In excellent storage conditions (i.e. amber bottles in a cool place with no air space) they will keep for about five years. Citrus oils tend to have a shorter shelf-life due to their high proportion of terpenes, as do absolutes and resins which thicken even more with age and the smell of the solvent becomes more noticeable.

Once essential oils have been diluted in a carrier oil, the shelf-life reduces dramatically. For maximum benefit use freshly made-up blends. A blend will keep for about three to six months if it is stored in an amber-coloured bottle in a cool place away from sunlight. If wheatgerm oil is added then the shelf-life is approximately six to nine months. If the smell alters and the vegetable oil becomes rancid then you should definitely discard it.

Dos and don'ts of buying and storage

- Clear glass or plastic bottles do *not* contain pure essential oils. Always buy oils in amber-coloured bottles.
- How old are the essential oils? When were they bottled?
- Are the oils in direct sunlight?
- Are the essential oils all the same price? If they are, then you are definitely not purchasing pure essential oils. For instance, pure essential oil of rose will be *far* more expensive then lavender or rosemary.
- Have the essential oils been diluted with any carrier oils? If so, when were they blended?

- Have the essential oils been adulterated with synthetic materials or bulking agents?
- Does the aromatherapy trader deal mostly with the perfume and food industries? Always look for an aromatherapy specialist.
- Does your supplier know about the essential oils?
- If blends are being sold, is there a qualified aromatherapist on the staff?
- Has the supplier been recommended to you?
- How long has the aromatherapy firm been established?
- Essential oils should always be kept away from young children. If they are taken internally some essential oils can be highly dangerous.
- Never leave bottled pure essential oils standing on plastic, polished or painted surfaces which can be damaged by the chemical constituents.
- Always store essential oils away from the naked flame.
- Store essential oils away from your homoeopathic medications which may be antidoted by the more powerful aromas.

Using essential oils

There are numerous ways in which essential oils can be used. I will outline some of the easiest and most effective techniques, but I urge you to be creative and fill your home with essential oils.

External Use

Baths

Aromatherapy baths have been employed for pleasure and therapeutic purposes throughout history. Hippocrates, the Father of Medicine, claimed that 'the way to health is to have an aromatic bath and a scented massage every day'. Baths were particularly enjoyed by the ancient Egyptians who had public baths, as did the Romans for whom they were an important aspect of social life. Water itself is therapeutic: 'water cures' are advocated by naturopaths, and various forms of hydrotherapy can be found in use nowadays at health farms and natural therapy centres.

Essential oils are simple to use in the bath. Just fill the bath and scatter about six drops of your chosen undiluted oil into the water, agitating it thoroughly. Do not add the essential oil until you have run the bath completely, otherwise the oil will evaporate with the heat of the water and the therapeutic properties will be lost before you climb in! Always disperse the oil – if you inadvertently sit down on neat essential oil of, say, tangerine you will jump up again very quickly! Shut the door to keep the precious aromas in and stay in the bath for at least fifteen minutes to allow the oil to penetrate deeply into your body tissues.

If you so desire, you may blend your six drops of essential oil with a teaspoon of carrier oil. This is particularly beneficial for those with dry skin, although carrier oils can leave a greasy ring around the bath. However, special, unscented bath oils, which contain natural dispersing agents, can be purchased. These leave the skin feeling soft but not greasy. Choose any vegetable oil such as sweet almond, wheatgerm, avocado or jojoba. You could mix up enough oil for several baths. Your skin will feel soft, nourished and supple.

Absolutes and resinoids such as **jasmine** and **benzoin** should be blended with a teaspoon of carrier oil as they tend to sink to the bottom of the bath and are difficult to clean off! I would strongly advise those of you with a sensitive skin *always* to blend the essential oil with a carrier oil. When using essential oils in a bath for babies and young children the oils should also be diluted. Undiluted essential oils can damage the eyes and babies and toddlers do have a tendency to rub their eyes. Use one drop in the baby's bath and two drops in a toddler's bath. I can endorse the effectiveness of this method.

Any essential oil may be added to the bath. Please exercise caution with the citrus oils and the stronger essences such as **black pepper** and **peppermint** if you have particularly sensitive skin. Just add three drops instead of six.

Hydrotherapy baths and Jacuzzis

Nowadays some people have their own Jacuzzi or hydrotherapy bath. Use the same number of drops as you would in a normal bath, although if it is a large hydrotherapy bath designed for two to three persons then ten drops may be added. Sprinkle in your essential oils after the bath has been filled.

The essential oils, however, must *not* be diluted in vegetable oils, which can coat the pipes.

Footbaths and handbaths

Footbaths and handbaths are highly beneficial in situations where it is impractical to enjoy a full aromatherapy bath – perhaps if you are elderly or have a disability. Footbaths, in particular, are incredibly relaxing at the end of a long, hard day. They are excellent for foot conditions such as athlete's foot and pain and swelling in the feet. Handbaths help to relieve the pain, stiffness and swelling of arthritis.

Add six drops of essential oil to a bowl of hand-hot water just before you immerse your feet or hands and soak for about ten to fifteen minutes.

Sitz baths and bidets

A sitz bath is invaluable in cases of cystitis, haemorrhoids, vaginal discharge, stitches after childbirth, and so on. Sprinkle about four to six drops of pure essential oil into a bowl of hand-hot water and sit in the bowl for about ten minutes. If you are fortunate enough to have a bidet then use the same number of drops. Ensure that the essential oil and water are thoroughly mixed.

Jug douche

This method is excellent for combating vaginal discharge and infections as well as anal problems. Boil a kettle and allow the water to cool in a one-litre jug ensuring that there is no limescale. Add six drops of essential oil. Lift both the seat as well as the lid of the toilet. Stand over the toilet and pour the solution over the vaginal and anal area. Dry the area gently.

If you wish to carry out this treatment at work you can prepare the solution in a one-litre plastic bottle.

Showers

A shower can never be as relaxing as a bath when using essential oils. However, it can be quite a stimulating way to begin your day.

Apply six drops of essential oil to a sponge or a flannel and rub all over your body towards the end of your shower. Alternatively, add your six drops of essential oil to two teaspoons of carrier oil and apply to your body before stepping into the shower. Make sure that you inhale the warming vapours.

Some essential oil suppliers stock shower gel to which essential oils may be added. (See 'Taking it Further' for information regarding suppliers.)

Compresses

Compresses can be used for a variety of disorders such as muscular aches and pains, bruises, rheumatic and arthritic pain, headaches and sprains.

You may apply compresses either hot or cold. Alternate hot and cold compresses are invaluable for treating sprains. As a general rule, where there is fever, acute pain or hot swellings use a cold compress. When treating chronic (long-term) pain use a hot compress.

To make a compress, mix approximately six drops of essential oil into a small bowl of water. Soak any piece of absorbent material such as a flannel, piece of sheeting or towelling in the solution ensuring that as much essential oil as possible is absorbed by your fabric. Squeeze out the compress so it does not drip everywhere and apply to the affected area. Wrap clingfilm around it or secure with a bandage. Leave for about two hours or even overnight. Where there is a fever replace with a new compress when necessary.

Gargles and mouthwashes

Gargles are particularly beneficial for sore throats, respiratory problems and loss of voice. After dental surgery gargling can help to relieve pains and inflammation, reduce blood flow and speed up the healing process. Gargle twice daily, although if the problem is acute then you can gargle every two hours.

Put two drops of essential oil into half a glass of water. Stir well, gargle and spit it out. *Do not swallow.* Stir again and repeat. Antiseptic oils such as **tea tree, sage, lemon** and **thyme** are excellent for treating sore throats. **Roman chamomile, geranium** and **sandalwood** will also soothe inflammation. **Myrrh** and **tea tree** combined are invaluable for treating mouth ulcers.

Inhalations

Inhalation of essential oils works upon the body, mind and spirit.

On a physical level there is a strong action on the mucous membranes of the nose, the lungs and the respiratory system in general. Conditions such as asthma, bronchitis, catarrh, coughs, colds, sinusitis and sore throats can all benefit enormously.

The inhalation of essential oils has a profound effect on the nervous system helping to relieve insomnia, anxiety and stress-related disorders, and lifting depression and negativity.

On a spiritual level some essential oils such as frankincense, cedarwood and linden blossom raise the consciousness and provide an excellent aid for meditation.

Steam inhalation

Add two to four drops of essential oil to a bowl of hot water. Cover your head with a towel and lean over the bowl inhaling deeply for one to five minutes. Keep your eyes closed to avoid irritation. If an asthmatic uses this method then just one drop is adequate. Take care with the hot water if there are small children around.

Water bowl

Put boiling water into a small bowl and add two to six drops of essential oil. Place the bowl on to a warm place, if possible, for maximum effect (e.g. a radiator). Ensure that small children do not drink the solution or knock it over. Close the doors and windows for a few minutes to enable the aroma to fill the room.

Handkerchief/tissue

Sprinkle a few drops of essential oil on to a handkerchief, paper towel or tissue and take a few deep breaths. This method is particularly effective for relieving nasal congestion and also for stopping panic attacks. Place the handkerchief in your pocket and you can continue to inhale the aroma throughout the day.

Hands

In a crisis situation put one drop of lavender on to your palm, rub your hands together, cup them over your nose and then breathe deeply. Avoid the eye area and ensure that your eyes are closed.

It is not a good idea to open a bottle of essential oil and inhale straight from it. Frequent opening of essential oils accelerates the rate of evaporation and therapeutic properties are lost. Also, removing essential oils stains from your carpet can be expensive!

Room spray

A room spray is a excellent way of purifying the atmosphere.
Add 250 ml of water to a plant spray and add 15–20 drops of
essential oil. Shake the bottle well and spray the room. You can
even spray carpets and curtains. Do *not* spray on to polished
surfaces.

Sprays can also be used to relieve irritation and pain as in
chicken-pox, shingles, burns and any infectious skin diseases.

Vaporisers and diffusers

Electric vaporisers are sometimes used in clinics and hospital
settings since they are considered to be safe. Electric diffusers,
which do not use heat, are also becoming popular. However,
both vaporisers and diffusers particularly can be rather
expensive.

Therefore, for home use, I recommend a clay vaporiser heated
by a night light. These are readily available. Put a few teaspoons
of water into the loose bowl on top and sprinkle two to six
drops of essential oil into it. Light the night light and the oil will
diffuse into the air.

Pillow and nightwear method

Place a few drops of essential oil on to a pillow or your
nightwear for relief from insomnia and to encourage easier and
deeper breathing. If desired, you could put the drops on to a
piece of cotton wool and place it inside the pillow case.

Light bulb ring

Two drops of essential oil can be sprinkled on to a ceramic or
metal ring which fits on to a light bulb. Only apply your oils
when the lamp is off and the ring is cool ensuring that you do
not get any oil on the light bulb itself or on the fitting, as
essential oils are inflammable.

Radiator fragrancer

Two to six drops of essential oil can be placed into a ceramic
container which fits on to a radiator by means of a magnet.

Alternatively, moisten a cotton-wool ball slightly with water,
sprinkle the drops of essential oil on to the ball and place it on
the radiator, or even lodge it by the pipe to avoid staining the
paint surface. The heat from the radiator will evaporate the
essential oil into the room.

Open fire

Put one drop of essential oil on each log before lighting the fire. As the logs heat up, the aroma will be released into the room. **Cypress**, **sandalwood** and **cedarwood** are particularly effective.

Candles

Add one to two drops of essential oil to the warm wax of a candle, taking care to avoid the wick since essential oils are flammable.

Massage

Massage even *without* essential oils is a powerful therapy (refer to my other book in this series, *Teach Yourself Massage* – see 'Further Reading'). The combination of pure essential oils and massage is even more potent. Massage is one of the most effective and beneficial treatment techniques. Essential oil constituents pass through the skin and they are taken into the bloodstream and can be carried to all the cells of the body.

Essential oils are not usually applied in an undiluted form to the skin except for emergencies such as burns, cuts or a sting. They must be blended with a suitable carrier oil in the appropriate dilution. You will find detailed descriptions of carrier oils in Chapter 4. When blending essential oil with a base oil, the essential oil content is usually between 1 per cent and 3 per cent. A massage takes between 10 ml and 20 ml of oil. Since a teaspoon holds approximately 5 ml, a treatment will require only two to four teaspoons of base oil. The following guidelines should help you (for babies please refer to Chapter 11 for appropriate dilutions):

> 3 drops of essential oil to 10 ml of carrier oil
> 4–5 drops of essential oil to 15 ml of carrier oil
> 6 drops of essential oil to 20 ml of carrier oil
> 15 drops of essential oil to 50 ml of carrier oil
> 30 drops of essential oil to 100 ml of carrier oil

Remember that if you are mixing up a large quantity (e.g. 100 ml) for daily use, then ensure that you add a teaspoon of wheatgerm oil to prolong the life of your blend. Oils which have been blended should be stored in amber-coloured bottles just like pure essential oils. If you wish to blend your essential oils into a vegetable-based lotion, rather than an oil, the dilution will be the same. Always label your bottles with the date and the oils which you have selected. When blending essential oils and base oils it is important to bear in mind that an increased concentration of essential oil does *not* imply that the formula will be more effective. Excessive amounts of essential oil will create unpleasant side effects and reactions. I would not advise you to put more than five essential oils together in one blend – usually two or three will be quite sufficient to create the desired therapeutic effects.

It is important to consider both the physical and emotional problems of the recipient of the treatment. Since many physical ailments stem from an emotional source, I strongly recommend the selection of at least one oil for any emotional imbalances. Remember that you are treating the whole person rather than the symptoms.

Always allow the recipient to smell the aromatic formula before you start the treatment. Rub a small amount on to the back of the recipient's hand. If the aroma is pleasurable then it will have a beneficial effect.

Ointments and creams

Sometimes you may prefer to apply a cream to a particular area of the body rather than an oil. It is possible to create some wonderful moisturisers for the face, and they make lovely presents. You can also blend your own hand creams and foot creams to alleviate cracked and chapped skin, redness and irritation, infections, chilblains, and so forth. Some aromatherapy suppliers produce a cream without essential oils to which you can add your own. Ensure that it is non-mineral based, organic and lanolin-free for optimum results (see 'Taking it Further' for information regarding suppliers).

You can, if you wish, prepare your own cream. You will need:

- yellow beeswax
- sweet almond oil (or avocado, jojoba or any vegetable oil)
- distilled water (or lavender water, orange water or rose water)

Use one part of beeswax to four parts of oil. A suggested recipe would be:

> 20 g of yellow beeswax
> 80 ml of sweet almond oil
> 40 ml of distilled water

Melt the beeswax and almond oil together in a pan of water over a gentle heat. Heat the distilled water gently in another bowl to blood temperature (37°C). Remove from the heat. Add the warm distilled water *gradually* to the oil mixture, beating all the time.

Once the cream has cooled you may add thirty drops of pure essential oil. Put the cream into amber-coloured glass jars and store in a cool place.

Internal use

Ingestion of oils is employed by some doctors in France and most of the research in France has been concerned with the internal use of essential oils. *All* the oil will be absorbed into the body via ingestion unlike inhalation and external application.

If essential oils are to be taken internally then *only* pure, high-quality oils should be used to avoid the risk of side effects. Absolutes and resinoids obtained via solvent extraction should *never* be ingested. Only distilled or expressed oils are recommended.

It is also very important to use exact and small doses – essential oils can be harmful and even dangerous in high doses. A safe dose is just two to three drops of essential oil to be taken three times a day. After three weeks stop taking the essential oils internally in order to rest the body and enable the liver to eliminate any toxic overload. As essential oils taste so powerful and bitter and can cause irritation they should be ingested in one of the following ways:

2–3 drops in a little red wine

or

2–3 drops in honey water (one teaspoon of honey to one-third cup of water) or in a spoonful of honey

or

2–3 drops in a dessertspoon of olive oil (extra virgin)

or

2–3 drops on a sugar lump

Take three times daily for no more than three weeks.

Aromatherapists do not prescribe essential oils for internal use, as their insurance does not cover internal use. However, many have used the above method effectively, with no side effects, for a long time. It is particularly good for treating sore throats and other respiratory problems, as well as for digestive problems such as indigestion and constipation, and urinary disorders like cystitis.

Do not give essential oils by mouth to babies or pregnant women.

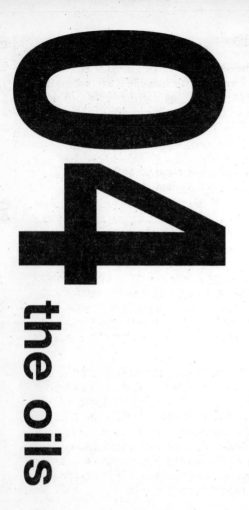

04

the oils

In this chapter you will learn:
- the properties and indications of a wide range of carrier oils
- the physical, mental, emotional and spiritual effects of 40 essential oils
- how to prepare and take the Bach Flower Remedies.

Carrier/base oils

Essential oils are highly concentrated in their pure state and they should not be used undiluted directly on to the skin. Therefore, a natural medium is required for an aromatherapy massage treatment. This medium is a vegetable, nut or seed oil which is referred to as the carrier, base or fixed oil.

The carrier oil chosen should be cold pressed. Oils produced by the process of 'hot extraction', although much cheaper, are unsuitable for use in aromatherapy as they are of an inferior quality. The base oil should be unrefined and untreated by chemicals. Vegetable oils have therapeutic properties in their own right and contain many vitamins and minerals, but the more highly processed the vegetable oils are, the less vitamin content will be retained. Colour and other additives may also be added at the oil pressing factories, which is also undesirable. For the purpose of aromatherapy always use cold pressed (preferably the 'virgin' type which is the first oil to be collected), unrefined, additive-free carrier oils. It is highly unlikely that you will find these oils on the shelves of your supermarket! Since the carrier oil is by far the largest part of any massage blend, always choose it carefully.

Mineral oil (purified, light petroleum oil) such as commercial baby oil, should *never* be used in aromatherapy as a carrier oil. Mineral oils tend to clog the pores whereas some of the vegetable oil molecules are absorbed through the skin. Mineral oils also do not have the nutritional constituents (vitamins, minerals and fatty acids) of the vegetable oils which nourish and benefit the skin. Mineral oil is used by the cosmetics industry because it does not become rancid. However, it stays on the skin like an 'oil slick' and prevents it from breathing.

The shelf-life of a base oil is dependent upon its fatty acid and vitamin E content. Vegetable oils which have a high proportion of saturated fatty acids will keep longer than those which are high in unsaturated fatty acids. The presence of vitamin E in the carrier oil will also increase the shelf-life.

Almond oil (sweet) – Prunus amygdalis

Sweet almond oil is probably the most common carrier oil used in aromatherapy. It is a yellow oil which is favoured by the beauty industry and is reputed to have been used by Napoleon's wife, Josephine.

Contents

Extracted by cold pressing from the kernels of the sweet almond, it is rich in vitamins including vitamin E and contains both monounsaturated and polyunsaturated fatty acids. Therefore, it has a reasonable shelf-life. If the oil is pale, it has probably been refined.

Properties and indications

It is useful for all skin types, although it is particularly indicated for dry, sensitive, inflamed or prematurely aged skin. It is also beneficial for relieving itching induced by conditions such as eczema.

Sweet almond oil is easily absorbed by the skin and it is not too heavy, thick or sticky. It also does not have a strong odour. It is highly recommended and may be used as a base oil 100 per cent.

N.B. Bitter almond oil which is highly toxic should *never* be used in aromatherapy.

Apricot kernel oil – Prunus armenica

Contents

Extracted by cold pressing from the kernel, apricot kernel oil is similar chemically to both sweet almond oil and peach kernel oil. Therefore, it is composed of both mono- and polyunsaturated fatty acids, vitamins and minerals. It is, however, more expensive than sweet almond oil as it is produced in smaller quantities. Some suppliers may try to sell sweet almond oil as apricot kernel or peach kernel oil, so make sure that you trust your supplier!

Properties and indications

It is suitable for all skin types especially dry, sensitive, inflamed and prematurely aged skin.

Although it may be used as a base oil 100 per cent it is usually added to a blend because of its enriching and nourishing properties. It is an excellent choice for a facial oil.

Avocado oil – Persea americana

This wonderful, dark, rich green carrier oil is cold pressed from the dried flesh of avocado pears which are not of a high enough quality for marketing as fresh fruit. If it has been refined, it will be a pale yellow colour. True avocado oil is quite difficult to obtain.

Contents

It is rich in lecithin, vitamins A, B and D and it contains both saturated and monounsaturated fatty acids. It has a long shelf-life.

Properties and indications

Avocado oil is a highly penetrative carrier oil and is invaluable for dry, dehydrated and mature skin. It is beneficial for eczema and the healing of wounds.

As it is a thick and viscous oil it is usually added to a blend in a 10 per cent dilution or less. However, it may be used in a higher concentration as a facial oil or where the skin is dry or damaged.

An avocado pear may be crushed and applied to the skin as a face pack to counteract dryness after a holiday where there has been too much exposure to the sun. (Avocado carrier oil is much less messy!)

Calendula oil – Calendula officinalis

Calendula oil is a 'macerated' oil (see page 14).

Properties and indications

It is renowned for its anti-inflammatory, healing and soothing properties and is highly beneficial for skin disorders. It can be included in preparations to protect against chapped or cracked hands and feet as well as chilblains. Calendula is useful for varicose veins, broken veins, leg ulcers and bed sores. It may help to reduce thread veins on the face if used over a long period of time. Cracked nipples in nursing mothers can be soothed by the application of calendula oil. It can also have a favourable effect on dry eczema. Scars may also be prevented or reduced. Calendula can also be applied gently to bruises.

Calendula oil would normally be added to a blend in up to 10 per cent solution, although it can be used in its own right. It is one of the expensive carrier oils.

Coconut oil – Cocos nucifera

Coconut oil has to be subjected to heat and refined in order to produce a workable oil. Although it can be used to aid tanning it is not really suitable for use in aromatherapy as a 'whole' oil. It is, of course, used a great deal for cosmetics, soaps and hair preparations.

Evening primrose oil – Oenorthera biennis

Contents

Evening primrose oil is cold pressed from the seeds. It is enriched with linoleic acid (a polyunsaturated fatty acid) and also contains gamma linoleic acid (GLA), oleic acid, palmitic acid and stearic acid.

Properties and indications

Heralded as a 'miracle of modern times', it has become increasingly popular to take evening primrose oil internally in capsule form for a whole host of conditions including premenstrual syndrome (PMS), menopause and other menstrual irregularities, high blood pressure and cardiac conditions, arthritis, eczema, psoriasis, allergies (particularly skin and respiratory problems such as asthma and hayfever), cystic fibrosis, diabetes, multiple sclerosis (MS) and Raynaud's disease. Evening primrose oil is even administered for psychological disorders such as schizophrenia and hyperactivity in children.

Externally it is excellent for dry, sensitive and allergic-type skin conditions helping to nourish the skin and calm down redness and irritation (e.g. eczema, psoriasis, dermatitis). Evening primrose oil counteracts and prevents premature ageing of the skin and it helps any skin condition aggravated by hormonal imbalances, such as acne at puberty and prior to menstruation, and also skin changes occurring at the menopause. There may also be an improvement in varicose veins. It makes a wonderful (albeit expensive) hair oil to be applied and left for a few hours prior to shampooing. Although evening primrose oil can be applied 100 per cent to small areas, it is normally used in up to a 10 per cent dilution.

Grapeseed oil – Vitis vinifera

I include grapeseed oil since it is widely used in aromatherapy and massage, although it is not one of my personal favourites. When I first began massage I was advised that it was a good general base oil, but I never did feel right about using it. As I am a person who follows her intuition I have not used grapeseed oil in my practice for many years.

Contents

Grapeseed oil is produced by hot extraction. It is almost colourless and odourless which may account for its popularity.

It contains vitamin E and also a high percentage of linoleic acid as well as other vitamins and minerals.

Properties and indications

Grapeseed oil can be used on all skin types but is particularly useful for oily skin. It is not 'sticky' and is easily and readily absorbed by the skin. It can be used as a base oil 100 per cent.

Jojoba oil – Simmondsia chinensis

Jojoba oil is not really an oil but is a liquid wax coming from Arizona, California and Mexico. This wax was discovered to have the same properties as sperm whale oil and it has taken its place in the cosmetics industry.

Contents

Jojoba is cold pressed from the nut which contains the liquid wax. It contains mystiric acid, protein and a waxy substance that mimics collagen.

Properties and indications

Jojoba is a yellow oil which is very stable. As it does not oxidise easily it does not become rancid. It has anti-inflammatory properties which makes it invaluable for red, inflamed conditions such as dermatitis, arthritis and swellings of all descriptions. It is a balancing oil and, therefore, all skin types from dry skin to oily skin will derive benefit. It can also be used in cases of acne, eczema and psoriasis.

Jojoba oil is marvellous for the face as it nourishes, moisturises and penetrates deeply. It is also used greatly in hair preparations. The wax content coats, protects and renews the hair. It helps damaged brittle hair and adds a shine.

Although jojoba oil may be used 100 per cent on small areas it is usually added in up to a 10 per cent dilution. It is an expensive carrier oil. However, a facial oil made of jojoba and essential oil can be compared favourably with any expensive cream.

Wheatgerm oil – Triticum vulgare

Wheatgerm oil is a rich orangey-brown colour and is usually added to a blend as it is considered by some to be antioxidant and, therefore, prevents the oils from becoming rancid. This is due to its high vitamin E content, making it an ideal preservative.

Contents

Wheatgerm oil is cold pressed. It contains vitamin E, protein, vitamins B_1, B_2, B_3 and B_6, zinc, iron, potassium, sulphur, phosphorus and linoleic acid.

Properties and indications

Wheatgerm oil is a rich and nourishing oil which is particularly good for dry, cracked and mature skin. It will improve itchy, flaky and peeling skin and, therefore, is beneficial in cases of eczema, psoriasis and sunburn. As it helps to prevent stretch marks, it is a must for the mother-to-be! Wheatgerm oil can also be valuable for hair care as it strengthens dry and brittle hair.

Wheatgerm oil is added in up to a 10 per cent dilution to preserve the life of a blend. However, it is too thick and heavy for use on its own and it has a strong smell of wheat.

N.B. Do not use in high dilution on individuals who have a wheat allergy.

The essential oils

There are hundreds of essential oils, although the experienced professional aromatherapist will probably use up to sixty. In this chapter I explore forty essential oils, outlining how each essential oil works upon the body and mind, as well as the spirit. For simplification I have included 'keywords' which indicate at a glance the main effects of each oil. Any precautions which must be observed are listed at the end of each essential oil.

Basil (French)/'True' Sweet Basil

Latin Name:	Ocimum basilicum
Family:	Lamiaceae (or Labiatae)
Method of extraction:	Steam distillation of the flowering tops of plant
Principal constituents:	Linalool, cineole, methyl chavicol
Origin:	France, Egypt, Italy, USA, Bulgaria, Hungary
Aroma:	Clear, spicy, sweet

Principal properties and indications – keywords

- Clarifying
- Decongestive
- Stimulating
- Strengthening
- Uplifting

Digestive system

Highly beneficial for relieving difficult and painful digestion, flatulence, gastric spasm, nausea and vomiting.

Muscles/joints

Relieves muscle spasms (cramp), gout, arthritis and rheumatism.

Nervous system

Probably one of the best nerve tonics. Basil uplifts, clarifies, strengthens and restores. Use for mental fatigue, inability to concentrate, nervous tension and depression.

Respiratory system

All respiratory problems including asthma, bronchitis, coughs, colds and whooping cough. Excellent for clearing the head. Use for catarrh, earache, nasal polyps, rhinitis, sinusitis, head colds, headaches and migraines.

Skin

Use as an insect repellent especially for wasps and mosquitoes.

Effects on spirit

Uplifting to the spirit, encouraging the opening of the 'third eye' and the development of intuition.

Special precautions

- Take care in pregnancy (although toxicity is unproven)
- Use in low dilution with sensitive skin (although sensitivity is rare)
- Do not use Exotic Basil also known as Comoran or Reunion Basil which has a higher methyl chavicol content.

Benzoin

Latin Name:	Styrax benzoin
Family:	Styraceae
Method of extraction:	Solvent extraction
Principal constituents:	Benzoic acid, vanillin conifery/ benzoate
Origin:	Sumatra Benzoin: Java and Malaysia. Siam Benzoin: Cambodia, China, Laos, Thailand and Vietnam
Aroma:	Vanilla-like

Principal properties and indications – keywords

- Comforting
- Gets things moving
- Healing
- Soothing
- Warming

Circulatory system

Stimulates the circulation and warms and regulates the heart.

Genito urinary system

Relieves all vaginal infections, discharges and irritations such as cystitis. Reduces fluid retention.

Muscles/joints

Helps arthritis, gout, rheumatism and fibrositis.

Nervous system

A warming oil that beings comfort to the recently bereaved and sad, lonely, depressed or negative individuals.

Respiratory system

Benzoin is a component of Friars Balsam and is invaluable for respiratory problems such as asthma, bronchitis, colds, coughs, flu, laryngitis and throat infections.

Skin

Excellent for cracked and chapped skin. Benzoin is an invaluable addition to any foot or hand cream. It soothes redness, irritation and dermatitis and encourages healing of sores and wounds.

Effects on spirit
Protects the spirit. Uplifting and invaluable for the heart and solar plexus.

Special precautions
- *Do not* take internally (it is not a distilled oil).

Bergamot

Latin Name:	Citrus bergamia
Family:	Rutaceae
Method of extraction:	Cold expression of the peel
Principal constituents:	Linalyl acetate, linalool, limonene
Origin:	Italy, Ivory Coast
Aroma:	Light, fresh, citrus

Principal properties and indications – keywords
- Antidepressant
- Antiseptic
- Balancing
- Uplifting

Digestive system
A tonic for the digestion stimulating a poor appetite and alleviating gas, colic and indigestion. Relieves halitosis (bad breath) when used as a gargle.

Genito urinary system
Has a strong affinity for this system helping cystitis, vaginal discharges, thrush and pruritis (itching).

Nervous system
Bergamot is a sedative yet uplifting making it ideal for all states of anxiety, depression and stress related conditions.

Respiratory system
Relieves sore throats, tonsillitis, colds, flu and all respiratory infections.

Skin
All stress related skin conditions improve such as eczema and psoriasis. Use for contagious conditions such as scabies, chicken-pox and head lice. Helps oily skin, acne, spots, boils and herpes.

Effects on spirit
Uplifting to the spirit, bergamot is excellent for the solar plexus and heart.

Special precautions
- *Do not* apply prior to sunbathing as it increases the photosensitivity of the skin due to its bergapten content, which accelerates sun tanning.

Black Pepper

Latin Name:	Piper nigrum
Family:	Piperaceae
Method of extraction:	Steam distillation of the dried, crushed black peppercorns
Principal constituents:	Mostly terpenes including caryophyllene, pinene, sabinene, limonene
Origin:	India, Indonesia, Malaysia, China, Madagascar
Aroma:	Sharp, spicy, hot, warming

Principal properties and indications – keywords
- Detoxifying
- Eliminative
- Get up and go
- Restorative
- Stimulant
- Tonic
- Warming

Circulatory system
A warming oil excellent for poor circulation, anaemia and after heavy bleeding.

Digestive system
Dispels toxins from the digestive system alleviating colic, constipation and food poisoning. Stimulates a poor appetite. Restores tone to the colon.

Muscles/joints
Restores tone to the skeletal system. Relieves muscular aches and pains, neuralgia, stiffness, arthritis, rheumatism, sprains and strains.

Nervous system
Can stimulate the mind aiding concentration and strengthening the nerves. Useful for coldness, indifference and apathy. May help impotence.

Respiratory system
Drives out coughs, colds, chills, catarrh and phlegm.

Effects on spirit
A grounding oil which also encourages change and instils positive thoughts and actions.

Special precautions
None.

Cajeput

Latin Name:	Melaleuca leucodendron
Family:	Myrtaceae
Method of extraction:	Steam distillation of the twigs and leaves of the tree
Principal constituents:	Cineole, limonene, pinene, terpineol
Origin:	Indonesia, Malaysia, Philippines, Vietnam, Java, South East Asia
Aroma:	Penetrating, medicinal odour

Principal properties and indications – keywords
- Antiseptic
- Decongestive
- Penetrating
- Stimulating
- Warming

Digestive system
Helpful for gastric spasm, upset stomachs and diarrhoea.

Genito urinary system
Cajeput alleviates all urinary infections such as cystitis and urethritis.

Muscles/joints
Excellent for pain relief. Use for all aches, painful joints, arthritis, rheumatism, gout, sciatica, sprains and strains.

Nervous system
Clears and stimulates the mind aiding concentration.

Respiratory system
Invaluable for the respiratory system as an inhalant and a chest rub, bringing down high temperatures and encouraging the expulsion of mucus. Use as a gargle for laryngitis and throat infections. Inhale for sinusitis and catarrh.

Skin
Use for oily skin, spots, boils and head lice.

Effects on spirit
Elevates the spirit and encourages the creation of new pathways.

Special precautions
- Take care with sensitive skin (although irritation unproven)
- Use in a low dilution.

Carrot Seed

Latin Name:	Daucus carota
Family:	Umbelliferae (or Apiaceae)
Method of extraction:	Steam distillation of the dried seeds
Principal constituents:	Carotol, limonene
Origin:	Europe
Aroma:	Sharp, pungent

Principal properties and indications – keywords
- Detoxifying
- Revitalizing
- Stimulating
- Tonic

Circulatory system
Stimulates poor circulation and purifies and detoxifies blood and lymph. Helps anaemia and boosts the immune system.

Digestive system
Alleviates constipation, irritable bowel syndrome, flatulence and liver problems. Aids digestion. Useful for eating disorders such as anorexia.

Genito urinary system
Helps fluid retention and cystitis. Carrot seed also regulates the menstrual cycle and balances the hormones.

Nervous system
Useful for confusion and indecision, carrot seed enables us to see situations more clearly. It stimulates and revitalises.

Skin
Invaluable for skin problems, it is a tonic increasing the elasticity of the skin. Useful for mature skins. It also helps reduce scarring, for instance after acne.

Effects on spirit
Beneficial for the 'third eye' and strengthens our inner vision.

Special precautions
None.

Cedarwood, Atlas

Latin Name:	Cedrus atlantica
Family:	Pinaceae
Method of extraction:	Steam distillation of the wood
Principal constituents:	Cedrene, atlantone, atlantol
Origin:	North Africa especially Morocco
Aroma:	Warm, woody, heady

Principal properties and indications – keywords
- Calming
- Detoxifying
- Peaceful
- Soothing
- Warming

Circulatory system
Excellent for poor circulation, blocked-up arteries (arteriosclerosis) and for boosting a clogged-up lymphatic system.

Genito urinary system
Eases vaginal discharges and infections. Recommended for fluid retention, burning pains and itching.

Nervous system
Beneficial for all states of nervous tension, instilling peace and tranquillity. Good for clogged-up individuals. A useful aid for meditation.

Respiratory system
Cedarwood helps to break up catarrh and expel mucus.

Skin
Helpful for cellulite, oily skin, acne and chronic conditions. It balances the production of sebum.

Effects on spirit
Cedarwood enhances spirituality and has an affinity for the crown chakra.

Special precautions
- Avoid when pregnant
- Do not use on babies and young children.

Chamomile (Roman) Chamomile (German)

Latin Name:	Anthemis nobilis/Chamaemelum nobile = Roman Chamomile
	Matricaria Chamomilla/recutica = German Chamomile
Family:	Asteraceae (or Compositae)
Method of extraction:	Steam distillation of the flower heads
Principal constituents:	75–80% esters including isobutyl angelate, chamazulene
Origin:	Great Britain, Hungary, Italy, France, USA
Aroma:	Warm, sweet, floral, aromatic

Principal properties and indications – keywords

- Balancing
- Calming
- Soothing
- Children

Circulatory system

Helps to relieve and prevent anaemia. Stimulates the white blood cells boosting the immune system. Reduces fever.

Digestive system

Alleviates difficult or painful digestion. Invaluable for children's problems such as colic and diarrhoea. Good for the liver.

Genito urinary system

All female disorders will respond especially when associated with nervous tension. Particularly indicated for menopause, PMS, painful or scanty menstruation.

Head

Relieves the pain of earache, headaches, migraine, toothache and neuralgia.

Muscular/joints

Useful for all aches and pains, arthritis, inflamed joints, sprains and strains.

Nervous system

A calming oil easing states of anger, irritability, restlessness and impatience. Excellent for combating insomnia.

Skin

Calms and heals hypersensitive, inflamed and allergic skin, eczema and psoriasis. Soothes burns and acne.

Effects on spirit

Calms the solar plexus.

Special precautions

None. A safe oil, suitable for babies, young children and highly sensitive individuals.

Clary Sage

Latin Name:	Salvia sclarea
Family:	Lamiaceae (or Labiatae)
Method of extraction:	Steam distillation of the flowering tops and leaves
Principal constituents:	Linalyl acetate, linalool
Origin:	Europe especially Russia, Britain, Morocco
Aroma:	Sweet, heady, floral

Principal properties and indications – keywords

- Euphoric
- Intoxicating
- Relaxing
- Tonic

Circulatory system

Excellent for reducing the blood pressure and counteracting palpitations.

Genito urinary system

Clary sage is often recommended for childbirth since it encourages labour yet promotes relaxation. It is a tonic for the womb and balances the hormones reducing PMS and relieves the pain of menstrual cramps.

Nervous system

A euphoric–sedative oil indicated for overactive and panicky states of mind. It induces a sense of well-being and optimism and creates a padding between you and the outside world. Very suitable for all stress related disorders and general debility whether physical, mental, nervous or sexual. It is invaluable for those endeavouring to withdraw from drugs.

Skin

Useful for soothing and cooling inflamed skin. It also helps to balance oily skin, dandruff, stimulates hair growth and prevents wrinkles from occurring.

Effects on spirit

Invaluable for balancing the solar plexus. It can also balance an overactive 'third eye'.

Special precautions

- Large doses should not be taken together with alcohol which may induce a narcotic effect.
- Some say avoid during pregnancy, although there is no research to support or reject this.

Cypress

Latin Name:	Cupressus sempervirens
Family:	Cupressaceae
Method of extraction:	Steam distillation of the needles and twigs
Principal constituents:	Pinene, carene, terpinolene, camphene
Origin:	Mediterranean area
Aroma:	Woody, balsamic

Principal properties and indications – keywords

- Astringent
- Fluid reducing
- Warming
- Tonic

Circulatory system
Renowned for reducing varicose veins and haemorrhoids.

Genito urinary system
Helpful for fluid retention and relieving menstrual problems, especially PMS and the menopause.

Nervous system
A comforting oil indicated for bereavement. Cypress relieves anger, irritability and all stress related conditions.

Respiratory system
Particularly indicated for spasmodic coughing such as whooping cough. Also relieves asthma and bronchitis.

Skin
Excellent for oily skin and for reducing excessive perspiration. Combats cellulite.

Effects on spirit
Helpful for coping with change and for finding your soul pathway.

Special precautions
None.

Eucalyptus

Latin Name:	Eucalyptus globulus
Family:	Myrtaceae
Method of extraction:	Steam distillation of the leaves and twigs
Principal constituents:	Cineole, pinene, cymene
Origin:	Australia, China, Portugal, Spain
Aroma:	Fresh, camphor-like, penetrating

Principal properties and indications – keywords
- Antiseptic
- Expectorant
- Stimulant

Circulatory system
Useful for poor circulation.

Genito urinary system
Excellent for all urinary infections, cystitis, thrush and to reduce fluid retention.

Muscular/joints
Excellent for all aches and pains, arthritis and rheumatism.

Nervous system
A stimulating oil which combats mental exhaustion and aids concentration.

Respiratory system
Invaluable as an inhalant and chest rub for all respiratory disorders. It decongests the head and chest and helps to expel mucus. Use for asthma, bronchitis, coughs, colds, flu, sinusitis and throat infections. It reduces fever, prevents the spread of infection and boosts the immune system.

Skin

Useful for infectious skin diseases such as chicken-pox and measles. Also for herpes, cuts and burns. An excellent insect repellent.

Effects on spirit

Encourages communication by opening up the throat chakra. May be useful for cleansing past traumas.

Special precautions

- A powerful oil not to be massaged into babies and very young children.
- Store away from homoeopathic medicines.

Fennel (Sweet)

Latin Name:	Foeniculum vulgare
Family:	Umbelliferae (or Apiaceae)
Method of extraction:	Steam distillation of the crushed seeds
Principal constituents:	Trans-anethole, methyl chavicol, fenchone
Origin:	France, Italy, Bulgaria
Aroma:	Aniseed-like, strong

Principal properties and indications – keywords

- Detoxifying
- Digestive
- Eliminative
- Energising
- Fluid reducing

Digestive system

Marvellous for cleansing the digestive system (and all other systems too) fennel relieves constipation, flatulence and nausea. An invaluable aid for slimming, curbing the appetite yet increasing energy levels.

Genito urinary system

Excellent for nursing mothers as it increases the flow of breast milk. Highly effective for the menopause since it encourages the body to produce its own oestrogen. Eases fluid retention.

Nervous system

Encourages the ability to see a situation clearly. Induces courage, strength and hope in the face of seemingly impossible hurdles. Fennel can help to curb addictions.

Respiratory system

Useful for bronchitis, flu and shortness of breath.

Skin

Indicated for toxic, congested skin, cellulite and bruises.

Effects on spirit

Helpful for clearing the 'third eye' chakra.

Special precautions

- Do not use bitter fennel
- Do not use excessively on young children or epileptics
- Avoid during pregnancy.

Frankincense

Latin Name:	Boswellia carteri
Family:	Burseraceae
Method of extraction:	Steam distillation of oleo gum resin of trees obtained as teardrops
Principal constituents:	Pinene, limonene
Origin:	Somalia, Ethiopia
Aroma:	Woody, spicy, balsamic, warming

Principal properties and indications – keywords

- Comforting
- Decongestive
- Expectorant
- Elevating
- Healing
- Rejuvenating

Genito urinary system

The bactericidal power of frankincense helps to combat cystitis. It is also useful for all vaginal discharges and is highly beneficial during the menopause.

Nervous system
Elevating yet soothing effect on the emotions. It allows past traumas and anxieties to fade away. Frankincense instils peace and calm and is an excellent aid for meditation. Useful for those who fear change.

Respiratory system
Ideal for asthma and other respiratory disorders, it has both physical and emotional benefits. Frankincense encourages the breath to slow down and deepen.

Skin
An excellent remedy for all types of skin. It rejuvenates and revitalises mature skin and wrinkles and helps to prevent ageing. Reduces scars and stretch marks.

Effects on spirit
Invaluable for achieving heightened states of spiritual awareness, opening up the crown and 'third eye' chakras.

Special precautions
None.

Geranium

Latin Name:	Pelargonium graveolens
Family:	Geraniaceae
Method of extraction:	Steam distillation of the leaves, stalks and flowers
Principal constituents:	Citronellol, geraniol, linalool, citronellyl formate, geranyl formate
Origin:	Reunion (Bourbon), Egypt
Aroma:	Sweet, rosy

Principal properties and indications – keywords
- Antidepressant
- Balancing
- Fluid reducing
- Healing
- Uplifting

Circulatory system
Helpful for varicose veins and haemorrhoids and effective for stopping bleeding.

Genito urinary system
Excellent for the menopause and PMS. It balances the hormones, reduces fluid retention and hot flushes and balances tension and depression. Helps cystitis.

Nervous system
Geranium is wonderfully balancing for the nerves dispelling anxiety, depression and nervous tension. May help infertility problems.

Skin
Very balancing for all types of skin – inflamed, oily, dry, combination and mature. Also helps eczema, dermatitis, burns, infectious skin diseases and cellulite. Excellent for head lice and as an insect repellent.

Effects on spirit
Invaluable for uplifting the spirit and calming the solar plexus and opening the heart.

Special precautions
None.

Ginger

Latin Name:	Zingiber officinale
Family:	Zingerberaceae
Method of extraction:	Steam distillation of the dried ground rhizomes
Principal constituents:	Zingiberene, β sesquiphellandrene, ar-curcumene
Origin:	India, China
Aroma:	Aromatic, hot, spicy

Principal properties and indications – keywords

- Digestive
- Fiery
- Pain relieving
- Stimulant
- Warming

Circulatory system

Highly effective for stimulating poor circulation and helps varicose veins and high cholesterol.

Digestive system

Excellent for all digestive problems especially nausea (travel, early morning sickness). Also for diarrhoea, constipation, hangover, indigestion, flatulence, loss of appetite and stomach cramps.

Muscles/joints

Indicated for all muscular aches and pains, arthritis, cramps, rheumatism, sprains and strains. Ginger works particularly well when these conditions are aggravated by damp.

Nervous system

A warming uplifting oil for counteracting coldness and indifference, apathy, lethargy and nervous exhaustion. Useful for weak-minded individuals. It also aids concentration and memory and boosts confidence.

Respiratory system

Excellent for coughs and colds. It helps catarrh, bronchitis and sore throats.

Effects on spirit

A grounding oil which brings balance to the chakras. Helpful for the 'third eye'.

Special precautions

Use in low dilutions if the skin is hypersensitive. At normal dosage no irritation will occur.

Grapefruit

Latin Name:	Citrus paradisi
Family:	Rutaceae
Method of extraction:	Cold expression of the peel of the fruit
Principal constituent:	Limonene
Origin:	California
Aroma:	Fresh, sweet, refreshing

Principal properties and indications – keywords

- Antidepressant
- Detoxifying
- Refreshing
- Uplifting

Circulatory system
Excellent for purifying the blood and for 'unclogging' the lymphatic system.

Digestive system
An excellent aid to digestion and for 'detox' diets. Useful for obesity, liver and gall-bladder problems.

Muscles/joints
Valuable for arthritis, gout, rheumatism. Also before and after exercise for preventing stiffness in the muscles and joints.

Nervous system
An uplifting effect on the mind, helping to lift depression and inducing euphoria. Helpful for dispelling bitterness and resentment. Beneficial for nervous exhaustion and stress relief.

Respiratory system
Helps coughs, colds, flu and glandular fever.

Skin
Useful for oily and congested skin, acne and cellulite.

Effects on spirit
Uplifts the spirits.

Special precautions
Take care with hypersensitive skin (although irritation is rare).

Jasmine

Latin Name:	Jasminum officinale
Family:	Oleaceae
Method of extraction:	Solvent extraction of the flowers
Principal constituents:	Benzyl acetate, benzyl benzoate, cis-jasmone, linalool, phytols
Origin:	Egypt, France
Aroma:	Exotic, floral, heady, sensual

Principal properties and indications – keywords

- Antidepressant
- Aphrodisiac
- Euphoric
- Healing
- Uplifting

Genito urinary system

In childbirth it helps to relieve pain, promote the birth and expel the placenta. It is very useful after childbirth since it stimulates milk production and prevents post-natal depression. A renowned aphrodisiac, jasmine can alleviate frigidity, impotence and premature ejaculation. It also increases the sperm count. Excellent for painful menstruation, PMS and the menopause.

Nervous system

A wonderful oil for problems of the nervous system, lifting sadness and depression and inducing optimism, confidence and euphoria. Counteracts apathy and indifference.

Skin

Excellent for all types of skin, jasmine increases the elasticity of the skin and reduces stretchmarks and scars. Also indicated for dry and sensitive skin.

Effects on spirit

Invaluable for the heart and solar plexus chakra. Excellent for stimulating the base chakra.

Special precautions

Do not take internally (it is an absolute).

Juniper Berry

Latin Name:	Juniperus communis
Family:	Cupressaceae
Method of extraction:	Steam distillation of crushed dried berries
Principal constituents:	Pinene, limonene, sabinene, myrcene, cymene, terpinene, terpinen-4-ol
Origin:	Eastern Europe
Aroma:	Fresh, woody

Principal properties and indications – keywords

- Antiseptic
- Cleansing
- Detoxifying
- Fluid reducing
- Purifying
- Tonic

Circulatory system

A wonderful detoxifier ideal for arteriosclerosis and a 'clogged up' lymphatic system.

Digestive system

Stimulates the elimination of toxins and therefore useful for obesity, constipation, stomach upsets after too much rich food and alcohol.

Genito urinary system

Excellent for relieving fluid retention and urinary infections such as cystitis. Use also for prostate problems, kidney stones and for scanty, irregular and painful menstruation.

Muscles/joints

An excellent remedy for arthritis, gout and rheumatic disorders, stimulating the elimination of uric acid and other toxins and relieving pain and stiffness.

Nervous system

An excellent oil for emotional depletion, clearing waste from the mind just as it does from the body.

Skin
Invaluable for cellulite, acne, blocked pores and oily skin. Also helps dermatitis, eczema and psoriasis. Since juniper encourages elimination, skin conditions may worsen before an improvement is seen.

Effects on spirit
A classic remedy for purifying and cleansing the spirit and for those who are unable to move on. Juniper helps to clear away the residues of unwanted past traumas.

Special precautions
- Avoid during pregnancy.
- Do not use excessively where there is inflammation of the kidneys.

Lavender

Latin Name:	Lavandula augustifolia/officinalis/vera
Family:	Lamiaceae (or Labiatae)
Method of extraction:	Steam distillation of the flowering tops
Principal constituents:	Linalyl acetate, linalool, terpineol, lavandulyl acetate
Origin:	France, Bulgaria
Aroma:	Sweet, floral

Principal properties and indications – keywords
- Antidepressant
- Antiseptic
- Balancing
- Calming
- Healing

Circulatory system
Excellent for high blood pressure, palpitations and all other cardiac disorders.

Digestive system
All digestive disorders especially in children, colic, diarrhoea, difficult and painful digestion, flatulence, indigestion, nausea and vomiting.

Genito urinary system

Helpful for cystitis, discharges and fluid retention. During childbirth lavender speeds up the delivery, calms the mother and purifies the air. Useful for PMS and the menopause.

Muscles/joints

All muscular aches and pains since lavender provides pain relief, relieves spasm and reduces inflammation. Arthritis, rheumatism, cramps, sprains and strains will all respond.

Nervous system

Lavender has a remarkably balancing effect relieving anxiety, depression, headaches and insomnia and encouraging calmness and serenity.

Respiratory system

As an immuno-booster lavender is recommended for protection against all infections, viruses, colds, coughs, flu, bronchitis, asthma and throat infections.

Skin

All skin care due to its powers of rejuvenation and balancing effects. Helps to heal bruises, burns, sunburn, acne, boils, eczema, fungal infections (e.g. athlete's foot), psoriasis, infectious skin conditions such as scabies and chicken-pox, wounds and sores.

Effects on spirit

Exerts a pronounced effect on the solar plexus, calming and soothing an angry spirit. Helps to balance all the chakras. May help to centre those on the wrong spiritual pathway.

Special precautions

None – lavender is used extensively on babies and children.

Lemon

Latin Name:	Citrus limonum
Family:	Rutaceae
Method of extraction:	Cold expression of the peel of the fruit
Principal constituents:	Limonene, pinene, terpinene
Origin:	Italy, Cyprus, Israel, California
Aroma:	Clean, crisp, fruity, refreshing, sharp

Principal properties and indications

- Alkaline
- Antiseptic
- Detoxifying
- Fluid reducing
- Purifying
- Tonic

Circulatory system

Stimulates and cleanses the circulatory system and boosts the immune system accelerating recovery time. Useful for high blood pressure, arteriosclerosis and for stopping bleeding.

Digestive system

Invaluable for the digestion relieving hyperacidity, stomach ulcers, liver and gall-bladder congestion. Good for obesity and detoxification.

Genito urinary system

An excellent diuretic relieving fluid retention. Also combats kidney and bladder infections and thrush.

Muscles/joints

Useful for arthritis, gout and rheumatism.

Nervous system

Stimulates a tired and exhausted mind encouraging clear thinking and aiding concentration.

Respiratory system

Relieves asthma, bronchitis, catarrh, colds, flu, laryngitis, throat infections and sinusitis.

Skin

Effective for cleaning out cuts and wounds. Reduces varicose veins and broken capillaries. Beneficial for ageing skin, brown patches, greasy skin, boils, herpes and scabies. May be applied neat to warts and verrucae.

Effects on spirit

Restores strength and vitality to a depleted spirit.

Special precautions

Avoid strong sunlight immediately after treatment.

Lemongrass (West Indian)

Latin Name:	Cymbopogon citratus
Family:	Gramineae (or Poaceae)
Method of extraction:	Steam distillation of fresh, partially dried leaves
Principal constituents:	Citral, geraniol, myrcene, methyl heptenone, nerol
Origin:	India, Guatemala
Aroma:	Lemony, sweet, strong, 'sherbet-like'

Principal properties and indications – keywords

- Astringent
- Refreshing
- Revitalising
- Tonic

Circulatory system

An excellent oil for stimulating the circulation. Invaluable for the immune system speeding up recovery time after debilitating illnesses such as glandular fever and M.E., and also for preventing illnesses from occurring.

Digestive system

Stimulates the appetite and useful for colitis, flatulence and difficult digestion.

Genito urinary system

Invaluable after childbirth for aiding post-natal recovery and promoting the flow of breast milk. Also useful for fluid retention.

Muscles/joints
Excellent for improving muscle tone. Relieves tired, achey legs and eliminates lactic acid. An ideal oil for sports people.

Nervous system
Refreshing and revitalising for the mind, it banishes apathy and lethargy and lifts depression. Indicated for nervous exhaustion.

Skin
A tonic for the skin. Indicated for open pores, excessive perspiration, acne, loose skin after dieting and cellulite. Use for infectious skin diseases such as scabies and measles. Excellent for fungal infections such as athlete's foot.

Effects on spirit
Uplifting for the spirit, encouraging change and growth.

Special precautions
Take care with hypersensitive skin.

Lime

Latin Name:	Citrus aurantifolia
Family:	Rutaceae
Method of extraction:	Cold expression of the peel of the unripe fruit
Principal constituents:	Limonene, linalool, camphene, cymene, myrcene, sabinene, citral
Origin:	USA, Italy, Central Mexico, West Indies
Aroma:	Refreshing, tangy, fruity

Principal properties and indications – keywords
- Refreshing
- Revitalising
- Uplifting

Circulatory system
An excellent oil for improving the circulation and balancing the blood pressure. Lime is a good immune booster and helps anaemia.

Digestive system
Lime stimulates a poor appetite and relieves heartburn and indigestion.

Muscles/joints
Beneficial for arthritis, gout and rheumatism.

Nervous system
An uplifting oil for those who are depressed or mentally run down. Recommended for apathy and lethargy.

Respiratory system
A most pleasant gargle for sore throats. Useful for asthma, bronchitis, catarrh, colds, coughs and flu.

Skin
Recommended for acne, boils, chilblains, cellulite, cuts and wounds, oily skin, mouth ulcers, warts and verrucae.

Effects on spirit
Lime opens up the heart chakra and clears the solar plexus.

Special precautions
Avoid strong sunlight immediately after treatment.

Mandarin

Latin Name:	Citrus reticulata
Family:	Rutaceae
Method of extraction:	Cold expression of the peel of the fruit
Principal constituents:	Limonene, terpenene, myrcene, cymene
Origin:	Italy, Spain, Greece, Brazil
Aroma:	Sweet, floral, tangy

Principal properties and indications – keywords
- Balancing
- Joyful
- Revitalising
- Uplifting
- Tonic

Therapeutic for young children, pregnancy and for people who are frail and elderly.

Circulatory system
A tonic for the circulation and for the immune system.

Digestive system
A gentle, calming tonic for the digestive system relieving flatulence and diarrhoea. Useful for stimulating a poor appetite following illness. Good for the liver and gallbladder.

Nervous system
Excellent for stress related disorders. Mandarin is uplifting, relieving depression and anxiety and it engenders feelings of joy and hopefulness.

Skin
A wonderful oil for the prevention of stretchmarks and reduction of scarring. A tonic for the skin. Helps oily skin and acne.

Effects on spirit
Encourages feelings of happiness in the heart chakra and balances the solar plexus.

Special precautions
Avoid strong sunlight immediately after treatment.

Marjoram (Sweet)

Latin Name:	Origanum marjorana
Family:	Labiatae
Method of extraction:	Steam distillation of the leaves and flowering tops
Principal constituents:	Terpinene, terpineol, myrcene, ocimene, sabinene, cymene, geranyl acetate
Origin:	France, Egypt
Aroma:	Sweet, warming

Principal properties and indications – keywords

- Calming
- Digestive
- Pain relieving
- Sedative
- Warming

Circulatory system

An excellent oil for improving the circulation. Marjoram regulates the heart and reduces high blood pressure.

Digestive system

Recommended for relieving constipation, diarrhoea, flatulence, indigestion, stomach cramps and ulcers.

Genito urinary system

Useful for alleviating painful and irregular menstruation. Helps to quell excessive sexual impulses.

Muscles/joints

Very effective for aches and pains, arthritis, rheumatism, sprains and strains. It alleviates pain, coldness and stiffness.

Nervous system

Marjoram has a warming and comforting effect on the emotions easing grief, sadness and depression and relieving all states of anxiety. Marvellous for those individuals who are unable to sit still.

Effects on spirit

Excellent for fearful individuals with much agitation in the solar plexus. Also for spirits who can find no peace and are constantly searching for the meaning of life. May also help detached individuals who find it difficult to be in this world.

Special precautions

Avoid during pregnancy (although adverse effects are extremely unlikely).

Melissa (Lemon Balm)

Latin Name:	Melissa officinalis
Family:	Labiatae
Method of extraction:	Steam distillation of the leaves and flowering tops
Principal constituents:	Caryophyllene, geranial, neral
Origin:	France, Republic of Ireland
Aroma:	Sweet, fresh, lemony

Principal properties and indications – keywords

- Antidepressant
- Sedative
- Soothing
- Uplifting

Circulatory system
Beneficial for high blood pressure and palpitations. It regulates the heart.

Digestive system
A gentle tonic for the digestive system helping indigestion, nausea, stomach cramps and liver problems.

Genito urinary system
Regulates the menstrual cycle and may help with problems of female infertility.

Nervous system
Wonderfully soothing for the nerves, dispelling depression, melancholy and insomnia. Use for shocks such as bereavement and also to counteract panic attacks and hysteria.

Respiratory system
Useful for asthma, bronchitis and coughs particularly if allergy or stress related.

Skin
Excellent for herpes. A cream with lemon balm which is sold in Germany is said to reduce the healing time and lengthen the time between attacks. Also helpful for allergies, wasp and bee stings.

Effects on spirit
Uplifting on the spiritual level with an affinity for the heart and solar plexus chakras.

Special precautions
Melissa is often adulterated with lemon, lemongrass or citronella. Take care with hypersensitive skins. Use in a 1% dilution (3 drops in 15ml carrier oil) or less.

Myrrh

Latin Name:	Commiphora myrrha
Family:	Burseraceae
Method of extraction:	Steam distillation of the crude myrrh
Principal constituents:	Curzerene, elemene, myrrh alcohols
Origin:	North Africa, Asia, especially Somalia, Yemen and Ethiopia
Aroma:	Warm, balsamic, musty

Principal properties and indications – keywords
- Antiseptic
- Anti-catarrhal
- Healing
- Rejuvenating

Digestive system
Relieves flatulence, diarrhoea, irritable bowel syndrome and haemorrhoids.

Genito urinary system
A cleanser of the womb, effective for thrush and vaginal discharges of all descriptions. Also helps with scanty and painful menstruation.

Nervous system
Helpful for weak-minded individuals who are apathetic, lethargic and difficult to spur into action.

Respiratory system
Highly effective for respiratory problems such as asthma, bronchitis, catarrh and coughs. Myrrh has a drying effect on mucus. Helpful as a gargle for sore throats and loss of voice and for mouth ulcers, infections and gum disorders such as gingivitis. It also stimulates the immune system.

Skin
Rejuvenates mature and wrinkled skin. Heals cracked, chapped and weepy skin. Combats fungal infections such as athlete's foot.

Effects on spirit
Beneficial for those who are 'stuck in a rut' and are unable to move on and grow. Helpful for those who see life as a series of negative obstacles.

Special precautions
Avoid during pregnancy (although there is no research to support or reject this).

Neroli (Orange Blossom)

Latin Name:	Citrus aurantium
Family:	Rutaceae
Method of extraction:	Steam distillation/solvent extraction of the freshly picked flowers
Principal constituents:	Linalool, linalyl acetate, limonene, geraniol, nerol
Origin:	Italy, Morocco, Tunisia, France
Aroma:	Fresh, floral, haunting

Principal properties and indications – keywords
- Antidepressant
- Aphrodisiac
- Sedative
- Stress and tension

Circulatory system
Excellent for high blood pressure, palpitations and false angina. Helpful for varicose veins.

Digestive system
Highly effective for colitis, chronic diarrhoea and nervous indigestion.

Genito urinary system
Excellent for the menopause and PMS.

Nervous system
Invaluable for all nervous problems, chronic and short term anxiety and panic attacks. It lifts depression and instils a feeling of euphoria. Relieves insomnia. Its aphrodisiac properties make it ideal for sexual problems such as impotence and frigidity caused by tension and apprehension.

Skin
A wonderful oil for all types of skin. It encourages the regeneration of skin cells and works wonders for mature skins. Recommended for preventing stretchmarks and reducing scars. Its gentle nature makes it ideal for sensitive skins.

Effects on spirit
Brings peace and tranquillity to a troubled spirit, and for those who repeatedly make the same mistakes in life. Especially beneficial for the solar plexus.

Special precautions
None.

Palmarosa

Latin Name:	Cymbopogon martinii
Family:	Gramineae (or Poaceae)
Method of extraction:	Steam distillation of the fresh or dried grass
Principal constituents:	Geraniol, linalool, geranyl acetate
Origin:	Madagascar, Brazil, Comoro Islands, Indonesia
Aroma:	Sweet, rosy

Principal properties and indications
- Rejuvenating
- Tonic
- Uplifting

Digestive system
Stimulates the appetite and is useful as a tonic for convalescence and appetite. Beneficial for anorexia.

Genito urinary system
Recommended as a uterine tonic and for assisting with childbirth. Useful for cystitis.

Muscles/joints
Excellent for relieving stiff muscles and joints, particularly following exercise.

Nervous system
A sedative yet uplifting oil ideal for releasing stress and tension. Raises self-esteem. Excellent for nervous exhaustion and as a tonic for the nerves.

Skin
Renowned for its beneficial effects on the skin. Useful for dry and cracked skin as well as acne since it regulates the production of sebum. Beneficial for mature skin and wrinkles as it aids cellular regeneration. Helps both dry and wet eczema.

Effects on spirit
Excellent for the solar plexus.

Special precautions
None.

Patchouli

Latin Name:	Pogostemon patchouli
Family:	Lamiaceae (or Labiatae)
Method of extraction:	Steam distillation of dried leaves
Principal constituents:	Patchoulol, pogostol, patchoulene
Origin:	Indonesia, India, Europe, USA
Aroma:	Sweet, earthy, musty

Principal properties and indications – keywords
- Antidepressant
- Healing
- Rejuvenating
- Soothing

Digestive system

Curbs the appetite and is useful for those who are trying to lose weight. Useful for relieving constipation, diarrhoea and irritable bowel syndrome. It gives tone to the colon and relieves bloatedness.

Nervous system

Popular in the 1960s possibly due to its ability to instil, peace, calm and love whilst at the same time helping to clarify problems. Beneficial for all stress related problems and sexual problems.

Skin

It encourages the regeneration of skin cells and is recommended for mature skin and scar tissue. Heals chapped and cracked skin and soothes and cools down skin redness. It also tones up loose skin after dieting. Fungal infections such as athlete's foot and allergies like eczema can also improve.

Effects on spirit

Exerts a grounding and balancing effect on the chakras.

Special precautions

None.

Peppermint

Latin Name:	Mentha piperita
Family:	Lamiaceae (or Labiatae)
Method of extraction:	Steam distillation of the leaves and flowering tops
Principal constituents:	Menthol, menthone
Origin:	USA
Aroma:	Cool, piercing, menthol

Principal properties and indications – keywords

- Cooling
- Digestive
- Pain relieving
- Stimulating
- Tonic

Digestive system
A powerful oil for all digestive problems, alleviating nausea and travel sickness, diarrhoea, constipation, indigestion and flatulence. Excellent for pain relief.

Head
Peppermint exerts a cooling and anaesthetic action on headaches and migraine. For toothache apply one drop neat on the affected tooth.

Muscles/joints
Invaluable for general pain relief relieving muscular aches, arthritis, neuralgia and rheumatism. One drop in a glass of water may be taken instead of aspirin.

Nervous system
An excellent oil for stimulating the mind, eliminating mental fatigue and encouraging concentration. In times of crisis peppermint strengthens yet numbs the nerves.

Respiratory system
Beneficial for asthma (especially food related), bronchitis, colds, coughs and flu.

Skin
Cools down sunburn and relieves itching and inflammation. Helpful for toxic, congested skin, acne and infectious skin conditions such as ringworm and scabies.

Effects on spirit
Peppermint will help to wake up, revive and stimulate the chakras into action. Also useful for a congested 'third eye'.

Special precautions
- Store away from homoeopathic medications and do not use in conjunction with homoeopathic treatment.
- Avoid using when breast feeding as it halts lactation.
- Take care with sensitive skins (although irritation is rare).
- Do not use on babies and young children.

Petitgrain

Latin Name:	Citrus aurantium
Family:	Rutaceae
Method of extraction:	Steam distillation of the leaves and twigs
Principal constituents:	Linalyl acetate, linalool
Origin:	France, Paraguay, Italy, Tunisia
Aroma:	Fresh, floral, bitter sweet. Reminiscent of neroli

Principal properties and indications – keywords

- Antidepressant
- Calming
- Soothing
- Tonic

Circulatory system

Valuable for stress related heart problems, it will slow down and regulate a rapid heart beat and dispel palpitations. It also stimulates the immune system.

Digestive system

Useful for calming the digestive system. Conditions such as nervous indigestion, diarrhoea and irritable bowel syndrome will respond.

Nervous system

Beneficial for all states of stress and tension. Petitgrain has a calming, balancing effect on the nervous system. It is also useful in convalescence.

Skin

Particularly suitable for oily skin and acne as it exerts a tonic and cleansing action on the skin.

Effects on spirit

Useful for the solar plexus chakra.

Special precautions

None.

Rose

Latin Name:	Rosa damascena (Damask rose)/ Rosa Centifolia (Cabbage rose)
Family:	Rosaceae
Method of extraction:	Steam distillation of the fresh petals (otto)/solvent extraction (absolute)
Principal constituents:	Stearoptene, geraniol, nerol, phenyl ethyl alcohol, citronellol
Origin:	Bulgaria, Morocco, Turkey, France, Italy
Aroma:	Sweet, heady, intoxicating, heavenly

Principal properties and indications – keywords

- Antidepressant
- Aphrodisiac
- Balancing
- Rejuvenating
- Uplifting

Circulatory system
Rose is very purifying for the blood and is an excellent tonic for the heart. It also reduces palpitations.

Digestive system
As a cleanser and tonic it is useful for constipation and liver problems.

Genito urinary system
This 'queen' of oils has a remarkable effect on disorders of the female reproductive system. It cleanses, regulates and tones the womb. PMS and the menopause will respond. Rose is a renowned aphrodisiac and is recommended for impotence and frigidity. It also aids conception and increases the production of semen.

Nervous system
The exquisite, luxurious aroma has a profound effect on the emotions alleviating grief, jealousy, resentment, stress and tension. It makes a woman feel feminine and positive. All states of depression may benefit from this oil.

Skin
Excellent for all types of skin especially dry, mature or sensitive. Rose calms down inflammation and reduces broken thread veins.

Effects on spirit
Particularly indicated for a closed heart chakra encouraging love and compassion. Releases past traumas.

Special precautions
None. Can be used safely with children. Do not take rose absolute internally.

Rosemary

Latin Name:	Rosmarinus officinalis
Family:	Lamiaceae (or Labiatae)
Method of extraction:	Steam distillation of the flowering tops
Principal constituents:	Cineole, pinene, borneol, camphor
Origin:	France, Spain, Tunisia
Aroma:	Clean, strong, slightly camphoraceous

Principal properties and indications – keywords
- Diuretic
- Pain relieving
- Restorative
- Stimulating

Circulatory system
Excellent for poor circulation and congestion in the lymphatic system. A good tonic for the heart, normalising blood cholesterol levels and arteriosclerosis.

Digestive system
Invaluable for many digestive complaints, particularly if detoxification is required. Use for constipation, flatulence, liver congestion, food poisoning and obesity.

Genito urinary system
Useful for combating fluid retention, discharges, cystitis and painful or scanty menstruation.

Head

Revives the senses of smell, speech, hearing and sight. A traditional ingredient of hair care preparations encouraging hair growth, relieving dandruff and combating head lice.

Muscles/joints

Highly recommended for pain relief in muscles and joints, easing arthritis, rheumatism and stiff, overworked muscles. Useful for poor muscle tone.

Nervous system

Activates and enlivens the brain, clearing the head and reducing mental fatigue. May help memory loss.

Respiratory system

Beneficial for asthma, bronchitis, catarrh, colds, flu and whooping cough.

Skin

Use for toxic, congested skin and infectious conditions such as scabies. Helps abscesses and boils. Reduces cellulite.

Effects on spirit

Excellent for 'loss' of spirit.

Special precautions

- Do not use extensively in the first stages of pregnancy (although side-effects are highly unlikely).
- Do not use extensively on epileptics.

Rosewood (Bois de Rose)

Latin Name:	Aniba rosaeodora / Ocotea caudata (Cayenne rosewood)
Family:	Lauraceae
Method of extraction:	Steam distillation of the wood
Principal constituent:	Linalool
Origin:	Brazil, Peru
Aroma:	Sweet, floral, woody

Principal properties and indications – keywords

- Balancing
- Rejuvenating
- Warming

Nervous system

A marvellous antidepressant, rosewood is a comforting and warming oil which has a balancing effect on the central nervous system. It clears the mind of clutter. Renowned as an aphrodisiac, it is valuable for frigidity, impotence and other sexual problems.

Respiratory system

Beneficial for colds, flu, viruses and throat problems. Rosewood soothes ticklish coughs. It also boosts the immune system.

Skin

Suitable for all types of skin – dry, oily, combination or sensitive. Highly rejuvenating for the skin combating prematurely aged skin and wrinkles.

Effects on spirit

Balances and enlivens all the chakras.

Special precautions

None.

Sandalwood

Latin Name:	Santalum album
Family:	Santalaceae
Method of extraction:	Steam distillation of powdered dried wood
Principal constituents:	Santalenes, santalols
Origin:	E. India
Aroma:	Sweet, warm, woody, lingering

Principal properties and indications – keywords

- Aphrodisiac
- Healing
- Soothing
- Uplifting

Circulatory system
A tonic for the heart, exerting a sedative yet regulatory effect.

Genito urinary system
Highly effective alleviating cystitis and vaginal infections of all kinds. Reduces fluid retention.

Nervous system
Renowned for its balancing effect on the nervous system, gently soothing away anxiety and tension. Reduces insomnia. An important aphrodisiac and therefore ideal for impotence and frigidity.

Respiratory system
Beneficial for chest infections, coughs, bronchitis and sore throats. It is antiseptic and boosts the immune system.

Skin
Sandalwood is used extensively for all skin complaints, especially dry, cracked and dehydrated skin. It makes a wonderful aftershave when blended with a carrier oil.

Effects on spirit
Brings peace and tranquillity to the troubled soul.

Special precautions
None.

Tea Tree

Latin Name:	Melaleuca alternifolia
Family:	Myrtaceae
Method of extraction:	Steam distillation of leaves
Principal constituents:	Terpinen-4-ol, cineole, terpinene
Origin:	Australia
Aroma:	Sharp, strong, medicinal

Principal properties and indications – keywords
- Antifungal
- Antiseptic
- First aid
- Stimulating

Circulatory system

A tonic for the heart stimulating the circulation and reducing varicose veins. Tea tree is a powerful immuno-booster and therefore may help to combat repeated infections, glandular fever and post viral syndrome myalgia encephalomyelitis (M.E.).

Genito urinary system

Excellent for cystitis, itching, thrush and vaginal discharges and infections.

Head

Ideal as a gargle for throat and gum infections, mouth ulcers and cold sores.

Nervous system

After an emotional crisis tea tree may be used to cleanse the shock.

Respiratory system

Beneficial for asthma, bronchitis, catarrh, colds, flu, sinusitis, and whooping cough.

Skin

A must for every household! Invaluable for acne, athlete's foot, boils, burns, cuts, herpes, itching, spots and sweaty or smelly feet. It may be applied neat to warts and verrucae.

Effects on spirit

Useful for shock if it gets stuck in the solar plexus and abdomen. Helps to eliminate old traumas.

Special precautions

None. Tea tree is often used neat for first aid purposes.

Thyme

Latin Name:	Thymus vulgaris
Family:	Lamiaceae (or Labiatae)
Method of extraction:	Steam distillation of the leaves and flowering tops
Principal constituents:	Thymol, cymene, linalool
Origin:	Europe, Israel, North Africa, USA
Aroma:	Strong, antiseptic, herbaceous

Principal properties and indications – keywords

- Antiseptic
- Energising
- Stimulant

Circulatory system

Stimulates the circulation and raises the blood pressure. An excellent booster of the immune system, extremely useful for convalescence. It also helps anaemia.

Digestive system

Cleanses the digestive system, improves constipation and restores the appetite.

Genito urinary system

Useful for fluid retention, urinary infections and vaginal discharges.

Muscles/joints

Recommended for sports injuries, gout, rheumatism and arthritis.

Nervous system

A reviving energising oil which stimulates the mind and improves the memory and powers of concentration.

Respiratory system

Helps asthma, bronchitis, catarrh, colds, coughs, sinusitis and throat infections. Excellent (as a gargle) for mouth and gum infections.

Skin

Useful for treating head lice and scabies.

Effects on spirit

Revives a tired spirit and helps to release blockages caused by past traumas.

Special precautions

- Avoid taking during pregnancy
- Take care with sensitive skins
- **Do not** use excessively in cases of high blood pressure
- **Do not** use on babies and young children.

Vetivert

Latin Name:	Andropogon muricatus / Vertivera zizaniodes
Family:	Gramineae (or Poaceae)
Method of extraction:	Steam distillation of the roots
Principal constituents:	Vetiverol, vetiverone, vetivene
Origin:	India, Indonesia, Comoro Islands, Java, Reunion
Aroma:	Earthy, smoky, woody aroma

Principal properties and indications – keywords
- Calming
- Protective
- Tranquillising

Circulatory system
Stimulates the circulation and acts as a tonic to the immune system.

Muscles/joints
A muscle relaxant, which helps to alleviate arthritis, rheumatism, cramps, sprains and strains.

Nervous system
Vetivert, 'oil of tranquillity', has a profoundly sedative effect and may be useful for those who are trying to stop taking tranquillisers or other addictive substances. Deep psychological problems may respond and hypochondriacs can benefit with regular use of this oil. Useful for insomnia.

Effects on spirit
Excellent for those who feel out of balance or ungrounded. Can also be used as a protective shield where individuals are oversensitive.

Special precautions
None.

Yarrow

Latin Name:	Achillea millefolium
Family:	Asteraceae (or Compositae)
Method of extraction:	Steam distillation of the flowering heads
Principal constituents:	Chamazulene, germacrene D, pinene, cineol, sabinene
Origin:	Indonesia, Germany, Bulgaria
Aroma:	Strong, medicinal

Principal properties and indications – keywords

- Anti-inflammatory
- Calming
- Sedative
- Soothing

Circulatory system

Lowers blood pressure and is a tonic for the circulation. Yarrow helps arteriosclerosis and varicose veins.

Genito urinary system

Excellent for the female reproductive system. Benefits irregular and scanty menstruation, painful, heavy periods, fibroids and prolapse of the uterus. Relieves bed-wetting, fluid retention and cystitis.

Muscles/joints

Excellent for inflammation. Yarrow helps rheumatoid arthritis, sprains and strains.

Nervous system

Yarrow exerts a soothing effect on the mind and is helpful for states of anger, impatience and irritability.

Skin

Recommended for oily scalp and skin, acne and inflamed skin conditions such as burns. May help baldness. Also good for eczema and psoriasis.

Effects on spirit

Valuable for protection.

Special precautions

- Take care in pregnancy.
- **Do not** use on babies and young children.

Ylang-ylang

Latin Name:	Cananga odorata var. genuina
Family:	Annonaceae
Method of extraction:	Steam distillation of flowers. The top grade (first distillation) is ylang-ylang extra which has a superior aroma to grades 1, 2 or 3
Principal constituents:	Linalool, caryophyllene, germacrene D, geranyl acetate, benzyl acetate, benzyl benzoate
Origin:	Comoro Islands, Madagascar, Reunion
Aroma:	Exotic, heady, sweet

Principal properties and indications – keywords

- Antidepressant
- Aphrodisiac
- Euphoric
- Soothing

Circulatory system

Reduces high blood pressure and has a regulatory effect on the heart. Reduces palpitations, rapid heartbeat (tachycardia) and rapid breathing (hyperpnoea).

Nervous system

A deeply relaxing oil releasing anxiety, tension, anger and fear. It uplifts depression and creates a sense of euphoria. Ylang-ylang relieves insomnia and thoughts that go round and round in the mind. A powerful aphrodisiac!

Skin

Used extensively for all skin care – both oily and dry skins benefit. It may also promote hair growth.

Effects on spirit

Excellent for the heart chakra and also for the solar plexus and base chakra.

Special precautions

None.

Bach Flower Remedies

The action of these Remedies is to raise our vibrations and open up our channels for the reception of the Spiritual Self; to flood our natures with the particular virtue we need, and wash out from us the fault that is causing us harm ... There is no true healing unless there is a change in outlook, peace of mind and inner happiness.

Dr Edward Bach

The thirty-eight Bach Flower Remedies aim to restore our balance and enable us to cope with the negative emotions that we experience and the problems that confront us in our everyday life. The Remedies are an excellent way to help ease the traumas that we face as we pass through the various stages of our lives.

They were created by the physician, Dr Edward Bach, who became disillusioned with the orthodox idea of treating symptoms with medicines that often had harmful side-effects. His system of healing is intended to treat the person and deal with the root cause of the problem rather than treating the disease. He firmly believed in the philosophy that a healthy mind ensures a healthy body: 'Take no notice of the disease; think only of the outlook on life of the one in distress.'

Bach began to search for the Remedies that would 'treat the patient not the disease' and discovered thirty-eight flowers which cover the many negative states of mind from which we can suffer. It is well known that persistent worry lowers the body's vitality and its natural resistance to disease so that physical illnesses such as colds, digestive disturbance and other more serious conditions are allowed to develop. If a patient's negative state of mind is treated (fear, depression, hatred, jealousy, guilty and so on) then restoring balance to the mind will restore balance to the body.

The Bach Flower Remedies are an invaluable accompaniment to the art of aromatherapy. I firmly believe that **every** aromatherapist should know how to use them. There are many parallels that can be drawn between essential oils and Bach Flower Remedies: it is as if they were made for each other. Essential oils are incredibly powerful on an emotional level, often bringing old, unwanted and buried emotions to the surface. The Bach Flower Remedies are absolutely ideal for coping with these states of mind. You will notice that when you read the chapters which concentrate on various conditions, I have indicated which Remedies could be used in combination with the aromatherapy treatments.

I have listed below a brief description of each of the thirty-eight Remedies. By far the best way to find out and remember what they do is to use them. There are numerous books on the market if you wish to learn more.

The thirty-eight Remedies

Agrimony for those who hide their mental torture behind a happy, smiling face

Aspen for fear of an unknown origin

Beech for those who are unable to tolerate other people's shortcomings

Centaury for the weak willed who find it impossible to say 'no'

Cerato for those who doubt their own judgement and constantly seek advice and reassurance from others

Cherry Plum for fear of losing one's mind and harming oneself and others

Chestnut Bud for those who repeatedly make the same mistakes

Chicory for those who are selfish, over-possessive and clinging

Clematis for those who are daydreamers, absent-minded and lack interest in the present

Crab Apple to cleanse the mind and body of anything which we do not like

Elm for those who at times are overwhelmed by responsibilities at work or home

Gentian for depression from a known cause and self-doubt

Gorse for those who are filled with utter hopelessness and despair

Heather for those who are totally self-centred, talking incessantly about their problems, leaving their listeners exhausted and depleted

Holly for envy, hatred, jealousy, suspicion and revenge

Honeysuckle for those who cling to the past, dwelling upon memories both happy and sad

Hornbeam   for that 'Monday morning' feeling

Impatiens   for impatience, irritability and restlessness

Larch   for fear of failure and lack of confidence

Mimulus   for fear of a known origin

Mustard   for black depression from an unknown cause

Oak   for those who struggle on in the face of adversity until they 'drop'

Olive   for those who are absolutely physically or mentally exhausted

Pine   for a guilt complex and self-reproach

Red Chestnut   for excessive fear and concern for others

Rock Rose   for terror, panic and extreme fright

Rock Water   for those who try to set the 'perfect example' for others and deny themselves the simple pleasures in life

Scleranthus   for indecisiveness and mood swings

Star of Bethlehem   to ease the after effects of a mental or physical shock

Sweet Chestnut   for those who suffer utter despair and are unable to see the light at the end of the tunnel

Vervain   for those who 'live' on their nerves and are incensed by injustice

Vine   for those who are domineering, strong, inflexible who take the leading role

Walnut   for change (e.g. teething, puberty, menopause) and for protection against outside influences

Water Violet   for those who are gentle and proud, preferring their own company

White Chestnut   for persistent, unwanted thoughts that go round and round in the mind

Wild Oat   for those who are unfulfilled and dissatisfied and cannot find their true pathway

Wild Rose   for apathy and resignation in life

Willow   for resentment and bitterness and feeling 'hard done by'

Rescue Remedy   is the most widely used of all the Flower Remedies and is for emergencies and traumatic situations; it contains five of the thirty-eight Remedies

Preparation and taking the Remedies

Bach Flower Remedies are completely natural and are extremely safe, producing no harmful side-effects. They may also be taken alongside all medications with no risk of conflict. You cannot overdose on them, and if an inappropriate Remedy is taken it will not cause any ill effects. The Remedies can be taken internally by people of all ages from babies to the elderly. Even pets and plants will benefit.

You may take a single Bach Flower Remedy or a combination of Remedies up to a *maximum* of six. To prepare a Remedy almost fill a 30 ml dropper bottle with pure spring water, add a teaspoon of brandy for preservation purposes and then add two drops of each of your chosen Remedies. Take four drops *at least* four times a day, either straight on the tongue or in some water. Drops may be added to a baby's bottle or if breastfeeding the mother should take the appropriate Remedies.

If a person is unable to take the drops orally, the Remedies may be applied to the lips, behind the ears, temples or wrists.

People often ask how long the Remedies take to act but there is no definite answer. Negative emotions which have developed recently should pass away fairly quickly, whereas deep-rooted problems will take longer to heal.

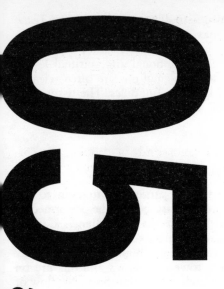

05

aromamassage

In this chapter you will learn:
- how to set the scene for an aromamassage
- the contraindications to an aromatherapy treatment
- how to perform a simple aromamassage.

Massage is a highly therapeutic tool in its own right (see *Teach Yourself Massage*). When massage is used in combination with the healing qualities of essential oils it constitutes a powerful therapy affecting the physical, emotional and spiritual levels. During an aromatherapy massage emotions are often released alongside the accumulated knots and nodules. The tissues and the nervous system are able to 'remember' both physical and emotional trauma.

Setting the scene

It is extremely important to pay particular attention to the environment in which the aromamassage is to be performed to derive maximum benefit from the treatment. Careful preparation and the right setting will make a good massage even better. Both the giver and the receiver should feel immediately relaxed. Always ensure that towels, cushions and oils are on hand so that you do not lose contact and thus break the flow of massage. An aromamassage should never be hurried.

Solitude and quiet

These are vital. Ensure that you choose a time when you will not be disturbed. Intrusions and distractions are extremely disconcerting, breaking your concentration and destroying the flow of your massage movements. Take the telephone off the hook and tell your friends and family not to enter the treatment room. You may decide to choose some soothing background music although this is a matter of personal preference. Some will prefer silence (see 'Taking it Further' for information on where to obtain massage/relaxation cassettes).

Cleanliness

This is essential. Always wash your hands before the treatment, as any stickiness will be instantly obvious to the receiver. Make sure that your fingernails are short – trim them as far down as possible. Do not wear any jewellery on your hands. Rings, bracelets and watches can all scratch the receiver.

Warmth

The room should be draught-free and warm yet well ventilated. Nothing will destroy an aromamassage more quickly than physical coldness: it is impossible to relax when you feel cold. The room in which you give the aromamassage should be heated prior to treatment and, as the receiver's body temperature will drop, ensure that spare towels are at your disposal. Keep all areas of the receiver's body covered, other than the part on which you are working. Warm your hands if they feel cold.

Lighting

Soft and subdued lighting will create the ideal atmosphere. Bright lights falling on the receiver's face will hardly induce relaxation and will cause tension around his or her eyes. Candlelight provides the perfect setting or you may wish to use a tinted bulb. Choose from pale pink, blue, green, peach or lavender.

Colour

The most therapeutic colours to have in the room are pastel shades – pale pink, blue, green or peach decor and towels are perfect for the occasion. Colours such as red will tend to create unwanted emotions like anger and restlessness.

Clothes

Wear comfortable and loose-fitting clothes as you need to move around easily and the room in which you will be working will be warm. White is the best colour to wear when giving an aromamassage since it will reflect any negativity which is released from the individual being treated.

Wear flat shoes or, even better, go barefoot. The receiver should undress down to whatever level he or she feels comfortable with. Suggest undressing down to the underwear. Point out that areas which are not being worked on will be covered up as this will create a sense of security and trust.

Finishing touches

Fresh flowers add a pleasant aroma to the atmosphere, or you can burn incense or essential oils prior to the treatment. Crystals may also enhance the environment. Rose quartz relaxes and soothes and amethyst is useful for absorbing negativity. You may put a drop of essential oil on to your crystals.

Equipment

Aromamassage surface

Work on the floor using a firm yet well-padded surface. This will allow you to give an aromamassage whenever you desire. Place a large, thick piece of foam, two or three blankets or a thick duvet on the floor. Use plenty of cushions or pillows during the treatment. When the receiver is lying on his or her back, place one pillow under the head and one under the knees to take the pressure off the back. When the receiver is lying on his or her front, place a pillow under the feet, one under the head and shoulders and perhaps one under the abdomen, if desired.

Ensure that you have something to kneel on to avoid sore knees. If you are unfortunate enough to suffer from back or knee problems it may be a good idea to invest in a portable couch. It is far less tiring and makes the receiver's body readily accessible. You could try improvising by using a kitchen table if the height is comfortable for you. Do not use a bed as most are far too soft and wide for massage purposes and any pressure applied is absorbed by the mattress.

Your attitude and state of mind

Posture

Whether you are working on the floor or at a table, keep your back relaxed yet straight throughout the aromamassage. When standing bend your knees slightly and tuck your bottom in so that your back can work from a secure base (i.e. the pelvis). Allow your thighs to do most of the work – not your back. Remember that it should be as relaxing to give a massage as it is to receive one. With practice you will learn to avoid tensing your muscles so that the healing energy can flow freely through your hands and body. If you do not pay attention to your posture you will become tired quickly. Habits are difficult to break so if you consciously control your posture now instead of slumping it will become automatic later on. Your shoulders, arms and lower back will thus take as little strain as possible. If you are using a couch, stand close to it so that you need to reach as little as possible.

Attunement

Your state of mind when giving an aromamassage is vital. The quality and success of a treatment depends upon having a calm state of mind. Do not attempt to give a treatment when you are feeling angry, moody, depressed or unwell. Your negativity will be transmitted. Your complete attention must be devoted to the receiver. If you are worrying about your own problems and your mind is drifting, this will be communicated immediately. Make sure that you are aware of the receiver's breathing and that you are sensitive to his or her reactions. Observe facial expressions and be aware of any tensing up in the muscles.

Spend time consciously relaxing yourself prior to the treatment and, most importantly, be guided by your own intuition. Take a few deep breaths before the aromamassage allowing all tension and anxiety to flow out of your body. Breathe in peace and breathe out love. Tune in to the person you are massaging. It may help to work with your eyes closed. Give yourself unselfishly to the massage.

Contraindications

As a general rule, most essential oils are safe provided they are used properly and sensibly. However, please observe the following at all times:

- Do not take internally;
- Do not apply essential oils to the skin undiluted (except for lavender and tea tree for first-aid purposes) as they are far too concentrated and can result in inflammation and allergic reaction;
- Keep oils away from the eyes;
- Keep the oils out of reach of children;
- Ensure that the dosage is accurate as too much essential oil can be harmful;
- Purchase only *pure* essential oils;
- Take care with particularly sensitive skins – it is possible to do a patch test if you are anxious;
- Do not massage where there is a high fever. The body has already raised itself to a high temperature to fight off the infection and does not need the burden of even more toxins to deal with. However, essential oils may be applied on compresses in order to reduce temperature;

- Do not massage the abdomen heavily during pregnancy, especially for the first three months where risk of miscarriage is at its highest. Beware of certain oils throughout pregnancy. Check that there are no special precautions for any of your chosen oils;
- Beware of infectious skin conditions (e.g. scabies), although aromatherapy baths and blended creams are recommended;
- Use only light pressure over severe varicose veins;
- Beware of recent scar tissue, open wounds and areas of inflammation;
- Beware of unexplained lumps and bumps – always have them investigated by a doctor;
- Avoid areas of inflammation (e.g. *bursitis* – 'housemaid's knee');
- Always dilute essential oils when adding them to a baby's or child's bath;
- Avoid exposure to strong sunshine or sunbeds immediately *after* an aromatherapy massage;
- Wait a couple of hours after a sauna: the pores are open as the body is still eliminating.

The treatment

Space does not permit me to describe a complete professional aromatherapy treatment. However, the following sequence will enable you to perform a few simple movements so that you can treat your family and friends. Obviously, if you intend to use aromatherapy professionally then you will need formal training which entails the study of specialised techniques too complicated to describe here (see 'Taking it Further' for reputable training establishments). Some of these techniques have been described in my Headway Lifeguide – *Aromatherapy*. Self-massage is described in detail in *Teach Yourself Massage*. Both books are published by Hodder & Stoughton (see 'Further Reading').

The back

Back aromamassage may be used to aid relaxation, and to relieve constipation, menstrual and respiratory problems. The receiver should lie on his or her front with one pillow under the feet, one under the head, and one under the abdomen if desired.

1 Start with both hands relaxed at the base of the receiver's back, one hand either side of the spine. Stroke both hands up the back using your body weight to apply pressure, spread your hands across the shoulders and then allow them to glide back gently. Repeat this movement as often as you like to promote deep relaxation.

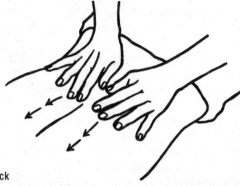

stroke the back

2 Starting at the base of the spine, make small, circular movements with your thumbs until you reach the neck (friction movements). Do not press directly on to the spine itself. Now perform these circular movements around each shoulder blade to loosen the knots and nodules.

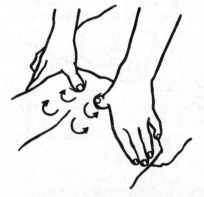

friction up the back from the base of the spine to the neck

3 Repeat step 1.

4 This movement is performed along the sides of the body and aims to drain away the toxins. Place both hands at the base of the spine on the side opposite you. Work up one side of the back pushing the toxins down towards the couch or the floor and gently flick them away. Repeat on the other side.

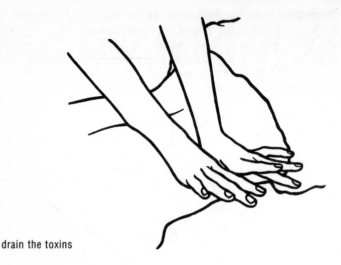

drain the toxins

5 To release tension from the shoulders work across the top of them alternately picking up and gently squeezing the tense muscles. This movement is called 'wringing' and if you are good at making bread this movement will come easily to you.

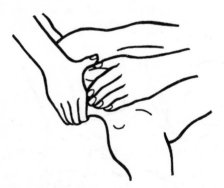

wring across the tops of the shoulders

6 To finish the back repeat step 1.

The legs

Aromamassage of the legs can be used to improve the circulation of the blood and lymph (to cleanse away toxins), relieve cramp, fluid retention and can prevent varicose veins.

1 Position yourself at the feet of the receiver. Beginning at the ankle stroke up towards the thigh with one hand in front of the other. Use no pressure on the way down.

2 To reduce tension from the muscles and to encourage the release of toxins accumulated in the deeper tissues, knead the muscular areas on the calf and thigh. Place both hands flat down and squeeze and pick up the muscles with alternate hands.

3 Repeat step 1.

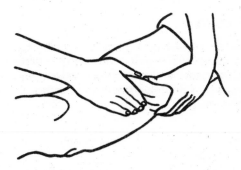

wring the thigh and calf muscles

The feet

Regular aromamassage of the feet can dramatically improve the circulation, relieve aches and pains and maintain flexibility and suppleness. It is wonderfully relaxing and soothing.

1 Stroke the foot firmly covering the top, sides and sole working from the ends of the toes towards the ankle. Slide around the ankle bones and glide back to your starting position.

2 Support the foot with one hand and use the knuckles of the other hand to circle firmly over the entire sole of the foot.

3 Repeat step 1 as many times as you like.

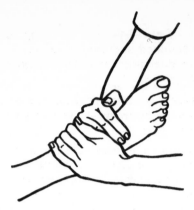

stroke the foot firmly

The abdomen

Aromamassage of the abdomen is excellent for relieving digestive and menstrual problems. It is easy to perform. Position yourself on the right-hand side of the receiver and massage in a clockwise direction circling around the abdomen with one hand following the other.

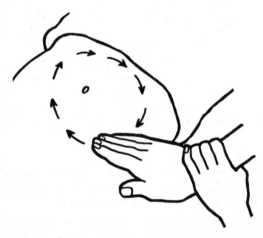

stroke the abdomen, working in a clockwise direction

The face

Aromamassage of the face is deeply relaxing and wonderfully uplifting. It can help to relieve skin problems, headaches, nasal problems such as sinusitis, slow down the ageing process and encourage clarity of thought.

1 Position yourself at the receiver's head and begin by stroking smoothly across the brow. Stroke outwards across the cheeks and then stroke outwards across the chin.

2 Place your thumbs at the centre of the forehead just between the eyebrows, press down quite firmly and hold for two seconds. Lift your thumbs and place them slightly further out along the brow bone and repeat the pressure. Continue until you have reached the outer corners of the eyes. Work the whole forehead as far as the hairline.

3 Repeat step 1.

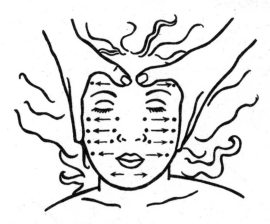

work across the face in strips using pressure points

4 Repeat step 2 on the cheeks and chin.

5 Spread out your fingers and thumbs and place the pads on the receiver's scalp. Circle them slowly and firmly, working gradually over the whole of the scalp area.

6 To complete your treatment stroke the hair from the roots to the tips and allow your hands to rest gently on the temples.

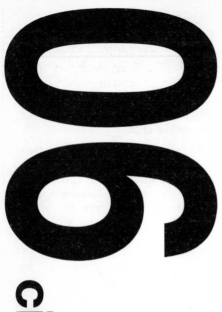

06

circulation

In this chapter you will learn:
- the causes and effects of the most common circulatory disorders
- the orthodox treatment for these conditions
- which aromatherapy oils are indicated for circulatory disorders and why
- how dietary and lifestyle changes can help.

Anaemia

Anaemia is the most common blood disease and is characterised by a deficiency of the haemoglobin (iron-containing) component of the red blood cells. Since red blood cells carry oxygen from the lungs to the tissues of the body in exchange for carbon dioxide, anaemia can also be thought of as a lack of oxygen being transported to the tissues in appropriate amounts and a build-up of carbon dioxide.

Symptoms

- fatigue, lassitude and a tendency to tire easily
- shortness of breath especially on exercise
- dizziness/fainting
- disturbed vision
- loss of appetite
- pallor of the skin
- palpitations
- angina
- rapid pulse
- ankle oedema (swelling) in severe cases where heart failure develops

There are a number of varieties of anaemia, but for the purposes of this book I shall discuss only iron deficiency anaemia. This type of anaemia has three causes:

1 Blood loss as in menstruation and bleeding from the gastointestinal tract as in ulcers, hiatus hernia and cancer. Even slight losses of blood if they occur over a long period of time can lead to anaemia – 1 ml of blood contains 0.5 mg of iron. Studies in developed countries have found evidence of iron deficiency in 30–50 per cent of the population. Iron deficiency usually develops slowly;

2 Increased body requirements as in pregnancy and during periods of rapid growth and lactation;

3 Nutritional deficiency caused by poor diet, ignorance, lack of food or malabsorption.

In addition to the general features of anaemia, iron deficiency is also characterised by a sore, smooth, red tongue, dry, brittle, spoon-shaped nails, 'pins and needles' and difficulties in swallowing.

Treatment

Orthodox treatment

A laboratory analysis of the blood is performed and a course of iron tablets or occasionally iron injections will be recommended. It is vital that the underlying cause is found.

Aromatherapy treatment

The following essential oils are particularly indicated for the treatment of anaemia.

Black pepper is a stimulant of the spleen which is involved in the production of new blood cells. It is also a stimulating and warming oil, in general helping to alleviate the feelings of utter exhaustion always associated with anaemia.

Roman chamomile, geranium and **lemon** are useful where the cause of anaemia is found to be menorrhagia (heavy blood loss). They will help to reduce the heavy bleeding, particularly **lemon**.

Thyme is also invaluable in the treatment of anaemia. It is a powerful stimulant and is widely used when the body is working 'under par'. Thyme is excellent for combating fatigue and lethargy and it also helps to stimulate the appetite which is often so poor where anaemia is present. It also stimulates the production of white corpuscles thus strengthening the body's resistance to illness.

Baths

Take daily baths using one of the following combinations added to the bath:

2 drops black pepper		2 drops geranium
2 drops Roman chamomile	or	2 drops lemon
2 drops lemon		2 drops thyme

Inhalations

Sprinkle a few drops of black pepper, lemon or thyme on a tissue and inhale several times deeply, keeping the eyes shut.

Aromamassage

The following oils may be helpful:

2 drops Roman chamomile	2 drops black pepper	diluted in
	1 drop Roman chamomile	15 ml
1 drop geranium	or 1 drop lemon	of
2 drops lemon	1 drop thyme	carrier oil

Contraindications

Thyme should be avoided during pregnancy and if the skin is exceptionally sensitive. **Lemon** should not be applied prior to sunbathing.

Bach Flower Remedy

The Bach Flower Remedy **Olive** is particularly indicated where the individual feels utterly exhausted and even totally drained to the point of crying.

For feelings of helplessness, despondency, despair and negativity, **Gorse** is strongly recommended.

Diet

A diet high in iron-rich foods is recommended, particularly during menstruation and pregnancy. Foods rich in iron include liver, green, leafy vegetables, blackstrap molasses, dried apricots and other dried fruits, shellfish.

A supplement of vitamin C enhances the absorption of iron greatly. At least 1 g of vitamin C daily with meals is indicated. Iron absorption is inhibited by tea and coffee drinking immediately after meals and by antacids. These should, therefore, be reduced.

Angina pectoris

Angina pectoris is caused by a lack of oxygen reaching the heart muscle, usually as a result of coronary vessel arteriosclerosis. This creates an atheromatous plaque which narrows and eventually blocks the coronary artery, resulting in a decreased blood and oxygen supply to the heart tissue and creating the characteristic pain. Angina is usually brought on by exertion and relieved by rest and nitrate drugs. It is also precipitated by stress, anxiety, emotion and any other situations making demands upon the heart.

Symptoms

- Constricting pain in the centre of the chest often radiating to the left shoulder blade and arm, neck, throat or jaw.
- Dyspnoea (breathing difficulties), nausea, sweating and faintness.

Treatment

Orthodox treatment

Angina requires strict medical supervision. Drug therapy is indicated and if this fails, coronary artery bypass surgery may be carried out.

Aromatherapy treatment

The aims of aromatherapy are to reduce stress and improve the circulation.

Baths

Take daily baths with the addition of six drops of any of the following oils.

Benzoin, black pepper, garlic, geranium, ginger, marjoram and **rosemary** will help to improve the circulation.

Bergamot, Roman chamomile, clary sage, frankincense, jasmine, neroli, rose, sandalwood, vetivert and **ylang ylang** will alleviate tension.

Inhalations

Put a few drops of essential oils of **lavender** on a tissue and inhale deeply, keeping the eyes closed to reduce stress, anxiety and the panic related to an attack of angina.

Aromamassage

Regular massage treatment is of enormous benefit in cardiac conditions. Massage is advisable at least once a month. The following formulae are recommended or you may create your own formulae choosing from the list.

1 drop bergamot	1 drop frankincense	diluted in
1 drop clary sage	or 1 drop geranium	10 ml of
1 drop ylang ylang	1 drop marjoram	carrier oil

1 drop benzoin	1 drop bergamot	diluted in
1 drop ginger	or 1 drop ginger	10 ml of
1 drop neroli	1 drop neroli	carrier oil

Contraindications

Avoid **marjoram** in pregnancy, although adverse effects are highly unlikely. Avoid **bergamot** prior to sunbathing.

Bach Flower Remedies

The Bach Flower Remedy **Impatiens** is invaluable for alleviating states of anxiety, impatience and irritability. **White Chestnut** is excellent for those whose minds are constantly occupied with persistent worrying thoughts. **Star of Bethlehem** will help to take away the effects of shock and trauma which can precipitate or occur after an attack. **Mimulus** can be taken by those who are fearful that another angina attack may occur.

Diet

It is essential to eat a healthy diet if angina has been diagnosed. Avoid junk food as much as possible since it contains high levels of sugar and salt. Avoid all fried foods - try to steam or grill. Eat plenty of fresh fruit and vegetables. Saturated animal fats such as lard and butter have been linked with a high risk of heart disease and cholesterol levels. Extra virgin olive oil is excellent and it is interesting to note that in Mediterranean countries, where enormous amounts of olive oil are consumed, the incidence of angina is low. Essential fatty acids are thought to prevent heart disease. They are present in oily fish such as mackerel and herring as well as in seed and vegetable oils. Dietary fibre also appears to protect the heart, although more research is needed. It is present in all plant foods including cereals (especially oats) and vegetables, pulses, fruits, nuts and seeds. Garlic is excellent for thinning the blood and it should be eaten raw whenever possible.

Supplements which may be useful include Co-enzyme Q10 which is thought to enhance energy production within the heart. Studies show that CoQ10 deficiency is common in patients with heart disease. Magnesium reduces spasms in the coronary arteries and improves heart function. Garlic capsules are recommended (although raw garlic is preferable).

Obviously you should not smoke, and if you are obese then you should try to lose weight slowly and sensibly. Gentle, regular physical exercise is vital for a healthy heart. Try to take a twenty-minute walk daily.

Hawthorn extracts are also of great value to sufferers of angina and other heart diseases. Experimental studies reveal that **hawthorn** dilates coronary blood vessels thus improving the blood and oxygen supply to the heart.

High blood pressure (hypertension)

The World Health Organisation defines high blood pressure as a systolic pressure greater than 160 and a diastolic pressure greater than 95. Currently 90 to 95 per cent of all diagnosed hypertension is termed as 'essential hypertension' (i.e. the underlying mechanism is unknown). In the other 5 to 10 per cent the hypertension is secondary to another disease (e.g. kidney disease, drugs, pregnancies, hormonal problems).

Severe hypertension is a serious disorder (systolic pressure greater than 220 or diastolic pressure greater than 140) requiring emergency treatment before heart or kidney failure, cerebral haemorrhage or fits occur. High blood pressure is a fairly common disorder and the incidence increases with age.

Symptoms

- headaches
- visual disturbance
- ringing in the ears
- breathlessness and/or chest pain

Treatment

Orthodox treatment

Drug therapy involves the use of diuretics and/or beta-adrenergic blocking drugs and vasodilators. Antihypertensive medications are among the most widely prescribed. Unfortunately there can be side effects.

All patients with hypertension should change both their diet and lifestyle. If the guidelines suggested were followed, most individuals would see a reduction in blood pressure.

If hypertension is not controlled then it can lead to hardening of the arteries (atheroma), heart failure, coronary disease and strokes.

Aromatherapy treatment

Aromatherapy can have a profound effect on blood pressure, although it is essential that dietary and lifestyle changes are also made. Essential oils which encourage deep relaxation and stress reduction are particularly invaluable.

Baths

Daily baths with essential oils added are highly therapeutic. Particularly useful essential oils include **chamomile, clary sage, frankincense, geranium, garlic, juniper, lavender, lemon, marjoram, neroli, rose** and **ylang ylang**. Suggested combinations are:

2 drops lavender
2 drops marjoram
2 drops ylang ylang
} or

2 drops clary sage
2 drops frankincense
2 drops marjoram
} or

2 drops Roman chamomile
2 drops geranium
2 drops rose
}

If a cleansing, detoxifying action is required, for instance when dietary changes are being implemented, use two drops fennel, two drops juniper and two drops lemon.

Aromamassage

Aromamassage once a week is invaluable for reducing blood pressure. If massage is performed at regular intervals the effects are quite remarkable and blood pressure may be lowered for several days after a treatment. The massage should be gentle and soothing, always in the direction of the heart. Suggested formulae:

1 drop clary sage
1 drop frankincense
1 drop lavender
} or

1 drop marjoram
1 drop neroli
1 drop ylang ylang
} diluted in 10 ml of carrier oil

For a detoxifying aromatherapy treatment:

2 drops juniper
1 drop lemon
} diluted in 10 ml of carrier oil

Contraindications

Fennel should be avoided in pregnancy and should not be used excessively by epileptics. **Marjoram** should be avoided in pregnancy, although an adverse reaction is highly unlikely. Avoid strong sunlight after the application of **lemon**.

Bach Flower Remedies

Remedies for stress relief include **Rescue Remedy, Impatiens** and **Vervain**. For those individuals who fail time and time again to learn their lesson that stress is no good for them **Chestnut Bud** is an excellent choice.

Diet

The diet should be low in salt, sugar and saturated fats as the effects of these substances on blood pressure are well documented. As the public has become aware of the dangers of salt, purchases of table salt have decreased but it is also important to look for hidden salt in processed and prepared foods. Sugar is also hidden in many foods. Increasing dietary linoleic acid as found in vegetable oils in Mediterranean countries, where the incidence of hypertension is lower, has an enormous hypotensive action. Fatty red meat can also cause blood pressure to rise.

A wholefood diet emphasising fruit and vegetables and garlic is recommended, with plenty of dietary fibre, particularly oat fibre.

The link between obesity and hypertension is well researched, and weight reduction will cause a substantial reduction in blood pressure. Weight reduction is probably more effective than taking antihypertensive drugs.

Caffeine, alcohol and smoking should also be eliminated from the diet as far as possible. Evidence reveals that 200 mg of caffeine (approximately three cups of black coffee) produces a temporary rise in blood pressure. Too much alcohol produces a significant rise in blood pressure in some individuals. It is well documented that smoking contributes to hypertension. Garlic has excellent hypotensive qualities. You should consume several cloves (preferably raw) daily. Cayenne pepper is also anti-hypertensive. Use one teaspoon a day in your cooking if you do not suffer from stomach ulcers. High levels of lead in water have also been linked with hypertension – buy a good water filter.

Supplements which have been found to be useful include:

- calcium – 1 g per day
- magnesium – 500 mg per day
- vitamin C – 1 g per day
- vitamin E – 200 iu daily
- garlic capsules – although raw garlic is preferable

Stress reduction is vital and deep breathing exercises and regular aromatherapy treatments will help to alleviate anxiety enormously. Regular exercise also helps to reduce states of hypertension. Only undertake an exercise programme with the permission of your doctor.

The herbs **hawthorn berry** and **mistletoe** have a regulating effect on blood pressure but they should be used only under the guidance of a qualified medical herbalist.

Low blood pressure (hypotension)

Hypotension is far less common than hypertension and is regarded as far less serious. However, individuals with chronic hypotension are more prone to dizziness and fainting due to the blood supply to the brain being momentarily interrupted. They may also feel fatigued and cold. Hypotension can be caused by anaemia, hypoglycaemia (low blood sugar), malnutrition or an underactive thyroid.

Treatment

Orthodox treatment
Drugs are not administered in the United Kingdom for low blood pressure which is considered not to be dangerous.

Aromatherapy treatment
Essential oils such as **black pepper, hyssop, peppermint, rosemary, sage** and **thyme** may all be used to help elevate the blood pressure.

Baths
Daily baths with the following combinations of essential oils are excellent for stimulating the circulation and aiding hypotension.

2 drops black pepper		2 drops rosemary
2 drops hyssop	or	2 drops peppermint
2 drops rosemary		2 drops sage

Aromamassage

Stimulating massage will help to improve the circulatory system generally. Suggested combinations are:

1 drop black pepper ⎫
1 drop peppermint ⎬ or
1 drop rosemary ⎭

1 drop hyssop ⎫
1 drop sage ⎬
1 drop thyme ⎭

diluted in
10 ml of
carrier oil

Contraindications

Avoid **hyssop, sage** (first few months) and **thyme** in pregnancy. Do not use hyssop and sage excessively in epilepsy. Avoid **peppermint** if taking homoeopathic medication.

Bach Flower Remedies

Olive is useful for combating fatigue and **Hornbeam** is useful for those 'Monday morning' feelings. Personally, I have found **Scleranthus** to be useful.

Diet

Avoid junk food. A high-protein diet may be beneficial as are leafy green vegetables, soya products, wheatgerm and baked potatoes which may help to restore elasticity to the arteries and normalise blood pressure.

Supplements of **hawthorn berries** and **mistletoe** may be prescribed by a qualified herbalist but should not be taken without supervision.

Siberian ginseng may also normalise blood pressure.

Poor circulation

Poor circulation is one of the most common problems that I have come across. I estimate that at least 25 per cent of my patients also suffer from deficient circulation. This condition particularly affects the hands and the feet.

Symptoms
- tingling feet
- cramps in hands and/or feet
- leg ulcers
- skin problems
- memory loss

Treatment

Aromatherapy treatment

Essential oils are extremely powerful for stimulating the circulation, causing the capillaries to widen so that a greater volume of blood can flow through them. Particularly effective oils include: **benzoin, black pepper, eucalyptus, garlic, geranium, ginger, juniper, lemon, mandarin, marjoram, rosemary, sage** and **thyme**.

Baths

Any of the essential oils suggested above may be added to your bath (six drops). Footbaths and handbaths are also invigorating for the circulation. If you are brave, try plunging your feet into hot and cold footbaths alternately.

Aromamassage

Daily massage of the hands and the feet improves the circulation dramatically. Patients who have regular aromatherapy treatments often report vast improvements in circulation. Suggested formulae are:

| 1 drop black pepper
1 drop geranium
1 drop ginger | or | 1 drop juniper
1 drop marjoram
1 drop rosemary | or | 1 drop benzoin
1 drop black pepper
1 drop thyme | diluted in 10 ml of carrier oil |

Contraindications

Sage (first few months) and **thyme** should be avoided in pregnancy. Epileptics should avoid excessive use of sage. Do not use sage when breastfeeding.

Diet

A healthy diet is essential with plenty of garlic and a teaspoon of cayenne pepper sprinkled on to food daily. Supplements include:

- gingko biloba which improves the circulation to the head, feet and hands
- vitamin C – strengthens the capillaries
- vitamin E
- garlic capsules – although raw garlic is preferable

Other treatments

Exercise

Exercise is vital to improve circulation. Rebounding on a mini trampoline is particularly effective, as is skipping, although a brisk walk daily will suffice.

Reflexology

Reflexology is also excellent for improving poor circulation. For those who are unable to exercise it is particularly recommended.

Varicose veins

Varicose veins are dilated, tortuous veins in the legs affecting four times as many women as men. Nearly 50 per cent of middle-aged adults suffer from varicose veins, with the veins just under the skin of the legs most commonly affected. If the deep venous valves or the valves between the deep and superficial valves are incompetent then blood leaks from the deep system to the superficial resulting in variscosity.

Long periods of standing and/or heavy lifting, pregnancy, obesity, damage or genetic weakness of the veins or venous valves, and increased straining and constipation can lead to the development of varicose veins.

If the involved vein is near to the surface, varicose veins are considered not to be harmful, although cosmetically they are unsightly.

N.B. If a varicose vein ruptures it will cause severe bleeding. Apply pressure and raise the limb to stop the bleeding – *never* use a tourniquet.

Symptoms

- weary, heavy, aching sensation in the lower legs which increases as the day progresses, especially if standing up
- pain over the varices
- swelling of the ankle and itching skin (due to leakage of the red cells)
- pigmentation and ulceration of the skin
- leg cramps while lying down

Treatment

Orthodox treatment
Support stockings are prescribed and injections and various surgical procedures are carried out including 'vein stripping'.

Aromatherapy treatment
The main objective of aromatherapy treatment is to improve the general tone of the veins and to strengthen the circulatory system.

Baths
Cypress (in particular), **geranium** and **lemon** are the three essential oils that I usually select for the treatment of varicose veins. Other alternatives are **black pepper, garlic, ginger, juniper, lavender, peppermint, rosemary** and **sandalwood**. Take daily baths using one or a combination of the oils above – it may take many months before any improvement is evident. Suggested formulae include:

2 drops cypress
2 drops geranium   }   or   2 drops ginger
2 drops lavender   2 drops juniper }
                                   2 drops rosemary

Aromamassage
Perform aromamassage *extremely gently* over an area of varicose veins, effleuraging from the ankle to the thigh. Employ massage particularly *above* the affected area of the vein. You can add essential oils to a pure organic skin cream and apply this daily. Dab the cream gently on to the affected area. The following massage blends should help to prevent as well as to alleviate varicose veins:

1 drop cypress
1 drop geranium   }   or   1 drop cypress   }   diluted in
1 drop lemon   1 drop juniper   10 ml of
                                  1 drop lavender   carrier
                                                          oil/lotion

Contraindications
Avoid **lemon** prior to sunbathing.

Diet

A high-fibre diet is important for the treatment and prevention of varicose veins. Individuals who have a low-fibre diet, high in refined foods, have a tendency to strain during bowel movements which increases the pressure in the abdomen and obstructs the flow of blood up the legs. This increased pressure weakens the vein wall, leading to the formation of varicose veins and/or haemorrhoids. A high-fibre diet will ensure that the stools are soft and easy to pass without straining.

Include lots of garlic in the diet (especially raw) to improve the circulatory system. Eat plenty of fresh fruit, vegetables, legumes and grains, especially foods such as blackberries, blackcurrants, citrus fruits, cherries, pineapples, rosehips, strawberries, raw peppers and green leafy vegetables. The berries will help to reduce the fragility of the capillaries and increase the muscular tone of the veins.

Obviously you should avoid junk food as well as strong tea and coffee.

Supplements include:

- gingko biloba to improve the circulation
- vitamin C – strengthens the capillaries
- vitamin E
- garlic capsules – although raw garlic is preferable

Other treatments

Rest

Rest with your legs higher than your head for at least fifteen minutes every day to improve drainage and to alleviate the uncomfortable aching sensation. The best position is to lie on the floor with your legs and feet up on a chair.

Exercise
Avoid standing in one place for long periods of time. Walking, cycling and swimming are particularly suitable forms of exercise.

Oils for other circulatory disorders

The following essential oils may be applied, using any of the methods outlined in Chapter 03. Daily baths, footbaths or handbaths in combination with regular aromatherapy massage are particularly recommended.

Arteriosclerosis
Black pepper, garlic, ginger, juniper, lemon and rosemary.

Blood purifying
Cypress, eucalyptus, fennel, grapefruit, juniper, lemon and rose.

Chilblains
Lemon

Fever
Bergamot, black pepper, chamomile, eucalyptus, ginger, juniper, lavender, marjoram and peppermint.

Heart tonic
Benzoin, lavender, marjoram, melissa and rose.

High cholesterol
Garlic, geranium, juniper and rosemary.

Immune system booster
Chamomile, cajeput, lavender, lemon, niaouli, tea tree and thyme.

Lymphatic congestion
Black pepper, cedarwood, chamomile, cypress, fennel, geranium, juniper, lavender, rosemary, sage and thyme.

Myalgic encephalomyelitis (ME)
Bergamot, cypress, chamomile, lavender, lemon, rosemary, sandalwood, tea tree and thyme.

Palpitations
Chamomile, garlic, lavender, mandarin, melissa, neroli, rose, rosemary, thyme and ylang ylang.

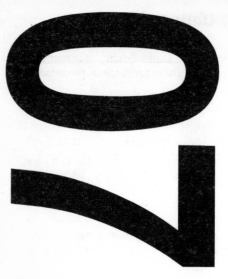

07

digestion

In this chapter you will learn:
- the causes and effects of some common digestive disorders
- the orthodox threatment for these conditions
- how aromatherapy may help and why
- how diet and lifestyle can relieve digestive problems.

Anorexia nervosa (and bulimia)

Anorexia is most common in teenage girls who become obsessed with their weight. Many sufferers are middle-class and of above average intelligence. Anorexia is on the increase and is now also affecting boys.

Symptoms

- persistent, active refusal to eat, sometimes accompanied by self-induced vomiting after food and laxative abuse
- alterations in body image – anorexics often wear loose clothing to hide their painfully thin frames
- amenorrhoea (loss of menstruation), slow pulse, decreased body temperature, loss of breasts, infertility
- constipation
- depressive, obsessional thoughts, low self-esteem, inclined towards perfection
- obsessions with various forms of exercise

Bulimia is a syndrome related to anorexia. The bulimic repeatedly binges on food and then induces vomiting.

Without treatment anorexia can be fatal.

Treatment

Orthodox treatment
Referral to a psychiatrist. Drug therapy such as antidepressants and tranquillisers. Admission to a hospital to achieve a target weight and, in severe cases, tube-feeding.

Aromatherapy treatment
When the anorexic can accept that treatment is required, aromatherapy can be highly successful. Psychotherapy or counselling should be used in conjunction with aromatherapy. The main aim of the treatment is to improve the psychological state of the anorexic. You must develop a trusting relationship if you are to make headway.

Baths
The following essential oils will help to alleviate depression, encourage optimism and improve self-esteem: **bergamot, chamomile, clary sage, frankincense, jasmine, lavender, neroli, rose** and **ylang ylang**.

Bergamot and fennel can be used to help regulate the appetite. Juniper will help cleanse the mind of the negative irrational thoughts and feelings of worthlessness. For courage try **black pepper, fennel, juniper, lavender, marjoram, melissa, myrrh, peppermint, rose, sage** and **thyme.**

For boosting energy levels and to combat feelings of being 'run down', **black pepper, peppermint, rosemary, sage** and **thyme** are invaluable.

Constipation can be treated with **black pepper, fennel, ginger, lemon, mandarin, marjoram, rose, rosemary** and **sage.** Suggested formulae:

3 drops bergamot 2 drops fennel 1 drop rose	or	2 drops black pepper 2 drops juniper 2 drops neroli	or	2 drops bergamot 2 drops mandarin 2 drops jasmine

Aromamassage

Perform aromamassage weekly. As the treatment progresses encourage the anorexic to employ some self-massage techniques. This is an excellent therapy and allows the sufferer to get in touch with his or her body and to learn to love and appreciate him or herself. It engenders a feeling of pampering and restores self-esteem and confidence. Suggested formulae:

1 drop bergamot 1 drop jasmine 1 drop rose	or	1 drop fennel 1 drop neroli 1 drop rose	diluted in 10 ml of carrier oil

For constipation the following formula is suggested and should be massaged into the abdomen in a clockwise direction.

1 drop black pepper 1 drop fennel 1 drop rose	diluted in 10 ml of carrier oil

Contraindications

Avoid **fennel, sage** (first few months) and **thyme** if pregnant. Epileptics should not use fennel or sage excessively.

Bach Flower Remedies

These Remedies are invaluable for treating the negative states of mind which surround the anorexic. **Gorse** will help to restore hope if the anorexic is totally pessimistic. **Crab apple** cleanses away feelings of ugliness, self-disgust, self-hatred and obsessions with body shape. It also reduces the hatred of food, and the feeling that food will contaminate the body. **Willow** is useful for those who feel that they are victims and who dwell upon their misfortunes. **Pine** is the remedy for the guilt and **mimulus** is to counteract the fear of eating. **Larch** is essential for restoring confidence. **Olive** is invaluable for boosting energy levels.

Diet

To gain weight the anorexic should eat small but frequent meals of nutrient-rich foods. Fruit and vegetables will probably not seem too much of a threat to the anorexic as they are regarded as 'slimming' foods. Nuts and other forms of protein are required to build up the body. Supplements of zinc help to restore the appetite and work on the psychological symptoms. Vitamin B complex, vitamin C, calcium and magnesium are also helpful.

Candida

Candida albicans, a type of yeast, is present in all of us. Normally the yeast lives harmlessly in the gastrointestinal tract (gut). However, if the yeast multiplies and overgrows it can migrate to the genito-urinary, endocrine, nervous and immune systems.

Symptoms

- thrush (of the vagina or mouth), bloating, flatulence, anal itching, altered bowel function (constipation and diarrhoea), heartburn
- headaches and migraine
- fatigue and lethargy
- depression, irritability, poor concentration
- allergies and low immune function
- PMS and other menstrual irregularities
- skin problems – acne, skin rashes, hives

The main cause of candida is prolonged antibiotic therapy which destroys the body's 'friendly bacteria' especially in the digestive tract, and promotes the overgrowth of candida. Oral contraceptives and corticosteroids also encourage the proliferation of candida. A person with low immune function is also more susceptible to the disease.

Treatment

Orthodox treatment
Anti-fungal drugs and pessaries will be prescribed.

Aromatherapy treatment
The following essential oils are highly effective for eliminating candida:

German chamomile, cinnamon, garlic, ginger, lavender, myrrh, patchouli, rosemary, tea tree, thyme and **yarrow.**

Baths
Daily baths or local applications are essential. You may need to continue these for a period of months before the candida is under control. Suggested formulae:

2 drops lavender 2 drops myrrh 2 drops tea tree	or	2 drops German chamomile 2 drops patchouli 2 drops tea tree	or	2 drops lavender 2 drops thyme 2 drops yarrow

The above essential oils may also be used in a sitz bath if the main problem is vaginal thrush.

Gargles
For oral thrush add one to two drops of any of the suggested oils to a glass of water and try to gargle several times a day.

Aromamassage
Although the local applications already described are invaluable, aromamassage is also recommended.

Perform abdominal massage to balance the constipation and diarrhoea. If constipation is the main problem then **black pepper, ginger, rosemary** and **thyme** may be used. If diarrhoea is present then try **chamomile, patchouli** and **yarrow.**

For headaches and migraines **chamomile, lavender** and **peppermint** will help to relieve the pain.

Tea tree, lavender, lemon, sandalwood and yarrow boost the immune system. The fatigue and lethargy which is so much associated with candida will respond to ginger, rosemary, tea tree and thyme.

Poor concentration and memory loss will benefit from essential oils of basil, peppermint and rosemary.

Yoghurt

1 drop German chamomile ⎫ added to a
1 drop myrrh   ⎬ carton of
1 drop tea tree   ⎭ 'live' yoghurt

Apply the yoghurt mixture to the vaginal area endeavouring to get it into the vagina. A tampon may be soaked in the yoghurt mixture and inserted into the vagina twice daily.

Contraindications

Avoid myrrh, sage (first few months) and thyme during pregnancy. Do not use sage excessively in cases of epilepsy. Avoid lemon prior to sunbathing.

Bach Flower Remedies

Olive is a remedy for extreme fatigue and lethargy. Crab apple is ideal for cleansing the candida fungus from the system. Mustard is helpful for bouts of depression and Impatiens soothes states of anger and irritability.

Diet

The diet should be free from all refined sugar, including fruit juices and honey, as candida thrives on high sugar levels. Avoid foods containing yeast or made with yeast, as well as any foods containing mould such as mushrooms and mouldy cheeses. Antibiotics should also be eliminated as much as possible under medical supervision.

Eat plenty of organic live, low-fat yoghurt which will regulate the friendly bacteria, and garlic and ginger which are antifungal. Cinnamon, rosemary and thyme also kill bacteria.

Supplements include acidophilis to replace the good bacteria and caprylic acid to inhibit yeast overgrowth. Iron and zinc may also be helpful.

Constipation

Constipation can be defined as the difficult or infrequent passing of motions. Some of the most common causes of constipation include:

- poor diet (high in refined foods and low in fibre) and inadequate fluid intake
- inadequate exercise or prolonged bedrest
- drugs – laxatives or enema (abuse), antibiotics, antacids, steroids, painkillers, antidepressants, diuretics

Treatment

Orthodox treatment

The doctor may prescribe laxatives or suppositories and may give advice on diet. Enemas are occasionally necessary.

Aromatherapy treatment

A large number of essential oils are helpful for the relief of constipation. These include: **black pepper, cardamon, cinnamon, fennel, ginger, juniper, lemon, marjoram, patchouli, rose, rosemary, sage** and **thyme**.

Baths

Daily baths with any of the oils suggested above will be beneficial.

Aromamassage

Aromamassage of the abdomen is by far the most effective aromatherapy treatment for constipation. Perform this twice daily where the problem is chronic; when the bowel has been retrained it can be performed whenever necessary. Commence at the bottom right-hand side of the abdomen working up the ascending colon using your three middle fingers to *gently* massage the colon. Use small, circular movements. Proceed across the abdomen to stimulate the transverse colon, and to complete your colon massage work down the descending colon to the left-hand side of the abdomen (you can perform these movements in the bath as well as with a massage blend). You should *never* experience extreme discomfort.

Some of the best combinations of essential oils are:

1 drop fennel 1 drop marjoram 1 drop rosemary	or	1 drop black pepper 1 drop marjoram 1 drop patchouli	or	1 drop cardamon 1 drop fennel 1 drop juniper	diluted in 10 ml of carrier oil

Although constipation may be caused by physical reasons such as poor diet and lack of exercise, bear in mind that it can be caused by emotional problems which have been suppressed. For these individuals, full body aromatherapy treatments are invaluable to encourage a 'letting-go' of all the emotional baggage and to reduce stress, anxiety and shock. The following combinations work on a physical, emotional and spiritual level:

1 drop juniper 1 drop marjoram 1 drop rose	or	1 drop bergamot 1 drop frankincense 1 drop rose	diluted in 10 ml of carrier oil

Contraindications

Do not use **fennel, marjoram, sage** or **thyme** excessively in pregnancy. Fennel and sage should be avoided by epileptics. Avoid **bergamot** prior to sunbathing.

Bach Flower Remedies

The Bach Flower Remedy **Crab Apple** is invaluable for cleansing and for anyone who feels disgust at bodily functions, dislikes themselves or considers themselves to be dirty or ugly. **Mimulus** can be used to help counteract the fear that passing a motion will be painful or that blood may be passed. **Agrimony** should be taken if an individual feels tortured and tormented inside. **Pine** is for the release of guilt and **Honeysuckle** is for letting go of the past. **Walnut** stimulates change and, therefore, helps to retrain the bowel.

Diet

Dietary changes are vital and you should eat a healthy, high-fibre diet to retrain the bowel. Dietary fibre increases both the frequency and quantity of bowel movements. Consume plenty of fruit and vegetables, as well as pulses, cereals, nuts and seeds.

Drink six to eight glasses of water daily. Never repress an urge to defecate, and you should never strain. You can use laxative herbs to re-establish bowel activity but do not abuse them. Cascara, cassia, senna, psyllium seed husks and aloe vera have long been used as laxatives. You can drink several cups of fennel and ginger tea daily to stimulate the bowel.

Regular exercise can also help to alleviate constipation. A brisk walk every day is ideal.

Heartburn/acid stomach/indigestion (dyspepsia)

The above conditions can be induced by a variety of factors:

- overindulgence in food and/or drink, rushing or not chewing food
- too much stress and tension which increases stomach acid
- an underlying disease – seek medical advice if symptoms persist

Symptoms

A burning sensation or discomfort behind the breastbone which may spread up the oesophagus to the back of the mouth.

Treatment

Orthodox treatment
Antacids will be prescribed and if symptoms persist, you may be referred to hospital for a barium meal.

Aromatherapy treatment
Dietary changes will be necessary but essential oils can provide relief from acidity and indigestion. Invaluable essential oils are: **basil, bergamot, black pepper, caraway, cardamon, chamomile, carrot seed, coriander, dill, fennel, garlic, juniper, lavender, lemon, marjoram, peppermint, rosemary, sage** and **spearmint.**

Compresses
A warm compress using one or a combination of the oils above can be comforting if placed over the stomach.

2 drops chamomile		2 drops cardamon
2 drops fennel	or	2 drops ginger
2 drops lemon		2 drops spearmint

You may also make up teas of dill, fennel, lemon, peppermint or spearmint. Place one drop of any of these essential oils into a glass of warm water to which you have added a teaspoon of honey. Another idea is to squeeze half a lemon into a glass of water.

Aromamassage

To alleviate the discomfort and pain, you may apply a blend of essential oils to the abdominal area, under the ribcage and around the throat area.

1 drop carrot seed		2 drops fennel		diluted in
2 drops dill	or	2 drops spearmint		10 ml of
1 drop ginger				carrier oil

If the indigestion is being caused by anxiety and worry, a different combination of essential oils are required:

1 drop chamomile		2 drops bergamot		diluted in
1 drop marjoram	or	1 drop rose		10 ml of
1 drop neroli				carrier oil

Contraindications

Avoid **fennel, marjoram** and **sage** if epileptic. Avoid **bergamot** prior to sunbathing. Avoid fennel and sage (first few months) if pregnant.

Bach Flower Remedies

Rescue Remedy can be taken to reduce stress and tension if this is the cause.

Diet

Eat slowly, chew thoroughly and try not to overeat too many heavy, rich meals. Try not to eat too many acid-forming foods which include biscuits, bread, cake, dairy foods, meat, pasta, sugar, alcohol, coffee and tea. Eat more alkaline-forming foods such as fresh fruit, vegetables and salad. Experiment with proper 'food combining' not mixing carbohydrate and protein together in the same meal.

Try to ensure that meal times are not stressful and not too late at night.

Obesity

Obesity is defined as a condition in which an individual's weight is 20 per cent or more above the ideal weight. It is a major problem in our society which affects approximately one-third of adults in Britain. This condition carries with it many adverse effects on health including reduced life expectancy, increased blood pressure, elevated cholesterol, risk of heart disease, late onset diabetes, digestive problems, arthritis and problems with the weight-bearing joints such as the knees or the hips. The obese individual also experiences much psychological trauma such as low self-esteem, depression, overeating for consolation and social rejection. Our society demands that we should be slim.

Although occasionally obesity is caused by disorders such as underactive thyroid, the majority of individuals are obese because they eat more than they need to maintain their normal level of activity.

Treatment

Aromatherapy treatment

We all over-indulge sometimes – Christmas is a prime example – and so essential oils that help us to lose weight are welcome. These include: **black pepper, cardamon, cypress, fennel, geranium, ginger, grapefruit, juniper, lemon, patchouli, peppermint, rosemary** and **spearmint**.

Fennel is probably the most useful oil for aiding weight loss and it has had a reputation of suppressing hunger since Roman and Greek times. Men ate fennel to give them energy and to allay hunger while on marches. Women ate fennel to prevent weight gain. Throughout the Middle Ages fennel was a permitted herb on fasting days. Fennel is a detoxifying oil and also an excellent diuretic and so helps to rid the body of any excessive fluids.

Black pepper and rosemary are powerful stimulants and tonics and, therefore, help to give the metabolism a 'kick start'. Juniper is a remarkable detoxifier and also is a diuretic. Cypress, grapefruit and lemon also help to cleanse the body and reduce excess fluid. Cardamon, peppermint and spearmint help the digestion.

After weight loss has been achieved the skin can become loose and saggy. Essential oils such as **black pepper, frankincense, lavender, lemongrass, mandarin, myrrh, patchouli** and **rosemary** may help.

Always consider the psychological state of the obese individual. Uplifting oils to improve self-esteem and to build up confidence and positivity are vital. The 'luxurious' oils such as **jasmine, rose** and **neroli** are particularly valuable. But if funds are low then **bergamot, chamomile, geranium, lavender** and **mandarin** are all beneficial.

Unfortunately essential oils will not miraculously dissolve away fat! They must, of course, be used in combination with a sensible diet.

Baths

Aromatherapy baths should be *preceded* by dry skin brushing. This will help to speed up the process of elimination and will unclog the pores of the skin and the lymphatic system. It will also improve the circulation. It should be performed at least once a day, brushing from the periphery of the body towards the centre and the heart. Suggested blends for the baths to encourage detoxification and to dispel fluid retention are:

2 drops cypress		2 drops black pepper		2 drops ginger
2 drops fennel	or	2 drops geranium	or	2 drops juniper
2 drops rosemary		2 drops lemon		2 drops spearmint

To uplift anxiety and depression:

2 drops bergamot
2 drops geranium
2 drops rose

Aromamassage

The use of aromamassage will help to change the way overweight people feel about themselves, encouraging a positive body image. Regular massage will also help to improve the appearance of the skin and stimulate muscle tone. A weekly full body massage is recommended paying particular attention to the 'problem' areas. Some blends which you can experiment with are:

2 drops bergamot	diluted		1 drop cypress	diluted in
1 drop fennel	in		1 drop ginger	15 ml of
1 drop rose	20 ml	or	2 drops mandarin	carrier oil
2 drops geranium	of carrier		1 drop peppermint	
1 drop juniper	oil			

Contraindications

Avoid **fennel** in pregnancy and in cases of epilepsy. Do not apply **bergamot** or **grapefruit** prior to sunbathing.

Bach Flower Remedies

Crab Apple is the remedy to improve self-image, cleansing away any thoughts of self-disgust and ugliness. **Larch** is indicated for lack of confidence. **Impatiens** is the remedy to help if there is impatience with slow weight loss. **Chestnut Bud** is for those individuals who have tried to diet many times before yet have reverted to their old ways. Chestnut Bud helps you learn from your past experiences. **Gorse** helps to engender hope and positivity.

Diet

A diet low in fibre, high in refined carbohydrates and fats is the main reason for obesity in the West. Avoid saturated fats such as in butter, lard and animal fats. Stop snacking on high-sugar foods such as biscuits, cakes and sweets. The diet should be high in fibre which tends to be filling, not fattening, and full of nutrients. Fruit, vegetables, salads, pulses and wholegrains are highly recommended. Drink dandelion, fennel or ginger tea to help weight loss.

It is important to combine a healthy diet with an exercise programme for optimum results. A brisk walk daily will suffice although swimming and cycling are also appropriate activities.

Try to be patient! If the weight loss is achieved gradually it is more likely to be permanent. If there is little or no decrease in weight during the first month, however, check with your doctor that you do not have a thyroid condition or another problem that makes weight reduction difficult.

Oils for other digestive disorders

The following essential oils may be applied, using any of the methods outlined in Chapter 03. Gentle massage of the abdomen and compresses are particularly effective for digestive disorders.

Colic
Basil, benzoin, bergamot, black pepper, caraway, cardamon, chamomile, cinnamon, clary sage, coriander, dill, fennel, frankincense, garlic, ginger, juniper, lavender, lemon, lemongrass, mandarin, marjoram, melissa, myrrh, peppermint, rosemary and spearmint.

Colitis
Bergamot, black pepper, cajeput, chamomile, coriander, fennel, garlic, juniper, lavender, lemongrass, neroli, peppermint, rosemary, spearmint and tea tree.

Diabetes
Eucalyptus, geranium and juniper.

Diarrhoea
Black pepper, cajeput, chamomile, cinnamon, cypress, eucalyptus, garlic, geranium, ginger, juniper, lavender, lemon, mandarin, myrrh, neroli, niaouli, patchouli, peppermint, rosemary and sandalwood.

Fistula (anal)
Lavender

Flatulence
Basil, bergamot, caraway, cardamon, carrot seed, cinnamon, chamomile, coriander, dill, fennel, ginger, lemon, marjoram, neroli, peppermint, rosemary, sage, spearmint and thyme.

Food poisoning
Black pepper, fennel, juniper, lemon and peppermint.

Gall bladder
Bergamot, carrot, chamomile, geranium, lavender, lemon, peppermint, rose, rosemary and ylang ylang.

Gastritis
Caraway, chamomile, lavender, lemon, melissa and sandalwood.

Gastro-enteritis
Basil, bergamot, cajeput, chamomile, fennel, garlic, geranium, lavender, peppermint, rosemary, spearmint, tea tree and thyme.

Hangover
Fennel, juniper and rosemary.

Hiccoughs
Basil, fennel and tangerine.

Liver
Carrot, chamomile, cypress, geranium, lavender, lemon, mandarin, peppermint, rose, rosemary, sage and thyme.

Loss of appetite
Basil, bergamot, black pepper, caraway, cardamon, chamomile, cinnamon, coriander, fennel, ginger, juniper, lemon, myrrh, peppermint, sage, spearmint and thyme.

Nausea/vomiting
Basil, black pepper, chamomile, fennel, ginger, lavender, mandarin, melissa, peppermint and spearmint.

Sluggish digestion
Black pepper, cardamon, coriander, fennel, ginger, juniper, peppermint and spearmint.

Spleen
Black pepper, chamomile, rosemary and thyme.

Stomach ulcers
Chamomile, garlic, geranium, lavender, lemon, peppermint, rosemary and spearmint.

Travel sickness
Lavender, ginger, peppermint and spearmint.

Worms and intestinal parasites
Bergamot, cajeput, caraway, eucalyptus, fennel, garlic, geranium, juniper, lavender, melissa, myrrh, peppermint, rosemary, spearmint, tea tree and thyme.

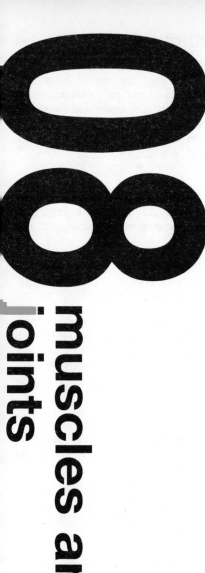

08

muscles and joints

In this chapter you will learn:
- the causes and effects of the most common muscular and joint problems
- the orthodox treatment for these disorders
- how aromatherapy may help and why
- how aromatherapy can be used in conjunction with dietary and lifestyle changes.

Arthritis – osteoarthritis

Osteoarthritis is a common degenerative disorder of the joints which occurs in almost everyone over the age of sixty. The average age of onset is fifty years. The principal joints which are affected are the weight-bearing joints (i.e. knees and hips) and the joints of the hands. The cartilage is destroyed, exposing the underlying bone and bony spurs called osteophytes are formed. It is the result of 'wear and tear'.

Symptoms

The main features are stiffness (especially in the morning), pain on moving the involved joint, limitation of movement and deformity.

Treatment

Orthodox treatment

Simple analgesics and non-steroidal anti-inflammatory drugs (NSAIDS) are prescribed. As these drugs are associated with side effects such as gastrointestinal upset, headaches and dizziness they should be used only for short periods of time. Joint replacement surgery is offered where there is serious degeneration.

Aromatherapy treatment

Aromatherapy is a highly effective treatment for this condition. It can reduce the pain of arthritis and also can improve and maintain the mobility of the joints.

Once again, aromatherapy must be used in conjunction with dietary changes. Start treatment as soon as possible in the early stages of the disease to achieve maximum effect.

Essential oils for arthritis include:

1 Analgesic (pain killing) oils: **angelica seed, benzoin, cajeput, Roman chamomile, eucalyptus, frankincense, geranium, ginger, lavender, marjoram, peppermint** and **rosemary**.
2 Detoxifying oils: **black pepper, cypress, fennel, ginger, grapefruit, juniper, lemon, rosemary, sage, thyme**.
3 Oils to improve the circulation: **benzoin, black pepper, eucalyptus, garlic, geranium, ginger, lemon, mandarin, marjoram, rosemary, sage, thyme**.

Baths

Aromatherapy oils should be added to your daily bath. Choose from the lists above or alternate the following arthritic bath formulae:

Warming and analgesic

1 drop benzoin
2 drops black pepper
1 drop ginger
2 drops marjoram

Detoxifying

2 drops cypress
1 drop fennel
2 drops juniper
1 drop lemon

If the arthritis sufferer has difficulty in getting into the bath then the same formulae may be added to a footbath or a handbath.

Compresses

These are excellent for providing pain relief. If the pain is acute then use a cold compress. For chronic pain use a hot compress or a combination of hot and cold. To make a compress mix six drops of essential oil into a small bowl of water. Soak a flannel or any piece of absorbent material into the solution. Gently squeeze the compress and apply it to the painful area.

Aromamassage

A full treatment will encourage the elimination of the accumulated toxins and improve the circulation with concentration on the particularly painful areas. The arthritis sufferer should gently massage the affected joints every day.

1 drop black pepper
2 drops frankincense
2 drops ginger
2 drops marjoram

or

1 drop eucalyptus
2 drops juniper
2 drops lavender
1 drop rosemary

diluted in
20 ml of
carrier oil

Contraindications

Do not use **fennel** and **sage** excessively in cases of epilepsy. Avoid **lemon** prior to sunbathing. Sage and **thyme** will raise the blood pressure.

Bach flower remedies

Use **Rescue Remedy** for pain relief.

Diet

It is vital that individuals with osteoarthritis are not overweight which puts stress and strain on the weight-bearing joints. Avoid refined carbohydrates and keep fats to a minimum. High-fibre foods are recommended. Plants in the deadly nightshade family can affect some arthritics (aubergines, tomatoes, peppers, tobacco and potatoes), so you could cut them out of your diet for a couple of months to see if there is any improvement.

Selenium ACE can be beneficial for osteoarthritis. Gentle exercise such as yoga is helpful for keeping the joints mobile.

Arthritis – rheumatoid (RA)

This is a chronic inflammatory condition that can affect the entire body although the joints most often involved are the hands, feet, wrists and ankles. Approximately one per cent of males and three per cent of females are affected in the UK and the average age of onset is 35 to 55.

What triggers this auto-immune reaction, where antibodies develop against components of joint tissues, remains unknown. Genetic susceptibility, lifestyle, diet and food allergies have been suggested.

Symptoms

The onset is usually gradual, beginning with mild fevers and vague joint pain. Joint symptoms often begin in the hands or feet in a symmetrical way. The involved joints are swollen, painful and stiff. Eventually joints become quite deformed.

Treatment

Orthodox treatment

Involves non-steroidal anti-inflammatory drugs (NSAIDS). As these drugs are associated with side-effects such as gastrointestinal upset, headaches and dizziness they should be used for short periods of time. Joint replacement surgery is offered where there is serious degeneration.

Aromatherapy treatment

Aromatherapy treatment can be successful, particularly if used in combination with dietary therapy since RA is not found in societies with a 'primitive' diet but is prevalent in those individuals consuming the Western diet.

Treatment should be directed towards reducing the inflammation as well as cleansing and detoxifying the whole body and alleviating pain.

Essential oils for rheumatoid arthritis include:

1 Anti-inflammatory oils: **celery, German chamomile, Roman chamomile, immortelle, lavender, myrrh, patchouli, peppermint, sandalwood, tagetes** and **yarrow**.
2 Cleansing oils: **angelica, black pepper, cypress, fennel, ginger, juniper, lemon, marjoram, rosemary, sage, thyme.**
3 Pain-relieving oils: **cajeput, Roman chamomile, eucalyptus, frankincense, ginger, lavender, marjoram, peppermint, rosemary.**

Baths

Footbaths and handbaths are invaluable for RA since this condition most often involves the hands and feet. Concentrate on using the anti-inflammatory oils during the 'flare-ups'. RA footbath/ handbath formulae (for inflammation):

3 drops chamomile (German/Roman) 1 drop immortelle 2 drops yarrow	or	2 drops chamomile (German/Roman) 2 drops lavender 2 drops peppermint

The above formulae may of course be used in baths.

Compresses

These are highly effective when placed on inflamed joints. Put three drops of chamomile and three drops of lavender/yarrow into a small bowl of water. Soak a piece of absorbent material such as a flannel into this solution. Squeeze it out and place it on to the swollen joint(s).

Aromamassage

A full treatment can be beneficial. However, perform only gentle stroking near any inflamed joints – just enough pressure to apply the oil. You can use aromatherapy treatments together – for instance, you can place compresses on the affected joints while other parts of the body are massaged. The following combinations may be useful:

Anti-inflammatory massage formula:

3 drops chamomile
(German/Roman) } diluted in 20 ml of carrier oil
1 drop immortelle
2 drops patchouli
2 drops yarrow

Cleansing massage formula:

1 drop angelica seed } diluted in 20 ml of carrier oil
2 drops black pepper
2 drops cypress
2 drops juniper
1 drop lemon

Analgesic massage formula:

1 drop frankincense } diluted in 20 ml of carrier oil
2 drops ginger
2 drops lavender
1 drop peppermint
2 drops rosemary

Contraindications

Sage and **thyme** raise the blood pressure. Do not use **fennel** and sage excessively in cases of epilepsy. Do not apply **lemon** prior to sunbathing. Avoid **peppermint** when taking homoeopathic medications.

Bach Flower Remedies

Rescue Remedy is useful for pain relief. **Agrimony** is for sufferers of RA who hide their pain behind a happy, brave face.

Diet

Since RA is found in societies consuming a Western diet, nutrition is an important factor. Food allergies can often be implicated in RA. It is well worth avoiding the possible culprits for a while. The most common foods are the nightshade family (tomatoes, peppers, aubergines and potatoes), dairy products and wheat.

The diet should be low in sugar, salt, refined carbohydrates and saturated fats. Eat lots of green vegetables, fruit and oily fish such as mackerel, salmon and sardines. If you have a juicer, carrot, celery and cabbage juices are beneficial.

Some RA sufferers benefit from fasting for a few days. Detoxifying oils should be used for this period.

Gout

Gout is caused by an increased level of uric acid, crystals of which are deposited in the joints. It is most common in men over the age of thirty and tends to run in families. Eating too much rich food and drinking too much alcohol may precipitate an attack. Trauma and some drugs may also cause it.

Symptoms

Gout is intensely painful and commonly affects the big toe which will be red, hot, shiny and incredibly painful. Subsequent attacks are fairly common.

Treatment

Orthodox treatment
Consists of the administration of anti-inflammatory drugs.

Aromatherapy treatment
This will involve using essential oils to combat the inflammation during the attack. Treatment will be aimed at preventing further attacks of gout and will involve detoxification and changes in diet. Individuals with gout are often obese and they will be encouraged to lose weight to avoid high blood pressure, heart disease and diabetes.

Essential oils for gout include: **angelica seed, basil, birch, cajeput, carrot seed, celery, juniper, lemon, rosemary** and **thyme**.

Baths
During an attack the affected joint should never be massaged. Footbaths are, therefore, particularly indicated and they can provide a great deal of pain relief.

Gout footbath formulae:

2 drops angelica		1 drop cajeput
2 drops carrot seed }	or	2 drops juniper
2 drops celery		1 drop lemon
		2 drops rosemary }

Compresses

The formulae recommended above can also be used to make a compress. Put the oils into a bowl of cold water, soak up with a flannel and place on the affected joint.

Aromamassage

The purpose of the aromamassage is to detoxify and thus maintain uric acid levels within the normal range. Any of the detoxification oils recommended for arthritis may be used. Two drops of each of juniper, lemon, rosemary and thyme is a good combination. If the sufferer is obese, refer to page 123 in this book for recommendations.

Contraindications

Thyme can raise the blood pressure. Avoid **lemon** prior to sunbathing.

Diet

Attention to diet is essential if gout is to be prevented. Avoid organ meats, red meat and alcohol in particular. Do not eat too much of the following: fats, refined foods, shellfish, yeast, cheese, salt, anchovies, coffee, tea and all foods and drinks containing sugar. If you are obese, it is vital to lose weight.

Drink plenty of water and eat lots of cherries. Other types of fresh fruit and vegetables are also beneficial. Supplements which may be helpful include celery seed extract capsules and vitamin C.

Oils for other muscular/joint disorders

The following essential oils may be applied, using any of the methods outlined in Chapter 03. Gentle massage of the affected area(s), in combination with daily aromatherapy baths, is recommended. Compresses are excellent for pain relief.

Aches and pains

Angelica, basil, bay, benzoin, black pepper, cajeput, caraway, chamomile, coriander, eucalyptus, frankincense, geranium, ginger, immortelle, juniper, lavender, lemon, marjoram, peppermint, rosemary, sage, tagetes, thyme, vetivert and yarrow.

Bruises
Black pepper, chamomile, fennel, geranium, ginger, lavender, marjoram, myrrh, peppermint, rosemary and sage.

Cramp
Basil, black pepper, cajeput, chamomile, cypress, lavender, marjoram, rosemary and valerian.

Lack of tone
Black pepper, juniper, lavender, lemongrass and rosemary.

Rheumatism
Bay, benzoin, black pepper, cajeput, caraway, cedarwood, celery, chamomile, coriander, cypress, eucalyptus, frankincense, ginger, immortelle, lavender, lemon, lime, linden blossom, marjoram, myrrh, peppermint, rosemary, sage, thyme, vetivert, violet and yarrow.

Sprains and strains
Bay, black pepper, chamomile, eucalyptus, ginger, lavender, marjoram, rosemary, sage, tagetes, thyme and yarrow.

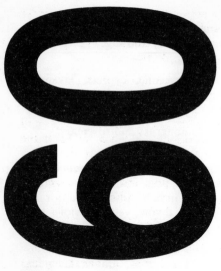

09

skin and hair

In this chapter you will learn:
- the main causes of skin and hair problems
- how to care for your skin and hair
- how to create individual blends for your hair and skin type
- simply dietary and lifestyle changes to promote healthy hair and skin.

Commercially-produced cosmetics contain synthetic substances such as preservatives, dyes and fragrances which are damaging to the skin's flora and protective 'acid mantle'. They promote ageing of the skin which results in wrinkles.

Commercial shampoos clean so thoroughly that the scalp's natural sebum is washed away. Because the scalp is thrown out of balance the hair is unable to grow as well as it should do. Shampoos also contain preservatives, chemicals, dyes and fragrances which can penetrate the hair follicles and enter the bloodstream. Ready-made cosmetics and shampoos also cost a great deal, far more than home-made natural cosmetics. Advertising and packaging are expensive and the manufacturer and the retailer also have to make a profit, of course.

Cosmetics made with essential oils can promote and protect your natural beauty and you know exactly what is in them. It is also satisfying and enjoyable to create your own aromatherapy products, and they do make wonderful gifts for your family and friends.

Skin

What causes skin disorders?

Skin problems can be caused by a variety of physical and emotional factors:

- poor diet
- deficiency of oxygen from closed, overheated rooms
- environmental pollutants
- chemical pollutants
- food intolerances (e.g. dairy foods, wheat)
- hormone imbalances
- smoking
- drugs
- synthetic cosmetics
- stress and emotional problems
- working or exercise outside in the sun, wind and rain

When tackling skin problems the only real long-term solution is to try to find out the root cause of the disorder rather than just working on the symptoms. A change in living and eating habits is often necessary alongside your essential oil régime. Our skin is a mirror of our inner health.

Dry skin care

Dry skin is lacking in moisture as the sebaceous glands are inactive and not producing enough sebum. Dry skin, unfortunately, is prone to more wrinkles than any other skin type. It needs to be 'fed' daily with nourishing and protective oils. Vegetable oils with essential oils are the best way to prevent the loss of moisture and to activate the sebaceous glands.

Dry skin base oils

Sweet almond, avocado, evening primrose, jojoba, apricot kernel and peach kernel oils are all excellent skin oil bases. Remember to add a small amount of wheatgerm oil to preserve your facial oil.

Essential oils for dry skin

Benzoin, carrot seed, Roman chamomile, German chamomile, frankincense, geranium, jasmine, lavender, neroli, palmarosa, rose, rosewood, sandalwood, vetivert, ylang ylang.

Suggested recipes for dry skin facial oils

You may select any of the essential oils from the list above and add them to your chosen carrier oil(s) or moisturising lotion. However, you may find the following recipes useful:

2 drops carrot seed			3 drops Roman chamomile	diluted in 30 ml of carrier oil
3 drops marjoram	2 drops rose		2 drops palmarosa	
3 drops rosewood	4 drops rosewood	or	3 drops rose	
2 drops fennel	4 drops sandalwood		2 drops rosewood	

Put all your ingredients into an amber-coloured bottle and shake well prior to use. Never use soap and water to cleanse your skin: this will cause further loss of moisture. Your facial oil will make a suitable cleanser.

Avoid hot facial steambaths and hot facial masks if you have dry skin. Use lukewarm compresses instead to cleanse and moisturise the skin.

Lukewarm compresses for dry skin

Heat up about a pint of water. Add four drops of essential oil and stir. Dip a face flannel into the solution and place it on your face until the compress cools off. The following recipes are recommended:

1 drop Roman chamomile		1 drop carrot seed
1 drop neroli	or	1 drop rose
1 drop rose		1 drop sandalwood

This skin type should also avoid all cosmetics containing alcohol which will strip even more moisture from the surface of the skin.

Diet

Eat plenty of fresh fruit and vegetables as well as lots of oily fish. Vitamin C, evening primrose oil and zinc may also help.

Try to avoid dry atmospheres and strong sunlight, wind and sunbeds. Do not smoke and drink excessively. Avoid stress.

Oily skin care

Oily skin occurs when the sebaceous glands produce too much sebum. The pores of the skin are often clogged and therefore have a tendency to form spots, blackheads and even acne. Areas particularly affected include the nose, chin and forehead. Oily skin is most common during puberty due to the hormonal changes which are occurring.

Facial steambaths and compresses are highly effective for oily skin. A facial steambath will cleanse the pores thoroughly, flushing out the toxic substances and stimulating the circulation. It should be carried out once a week.

Facial steambath for oily skin

Boil one to two pints of water and pour into a bowl. Add approximately six drops of essential oil. Bend your head over the bowl and cover your head with a towel. Steam your face for approximately ten minutes. Suggested recipes:

2 drops cypress		2 drops geranium	in a
2 drops lemon	or	2 drops rosemary	bowl of
2 drops juniper		2 drops tea tree	water

Face masks are also beneficial for oily skin. They cleanse, tauten and invigorate the skin. The most important ingredient of a face pack is fuller's earth or clay which will pull the toxins out of the skin.

Face mask for oily skin

2 tablespoons of clay/fuller's earth
1 teaspoon lemon pulp
1 teaspoon water
1 teaspoon honey
1 drop cypress
1 drop juniper

Mix the above ingredients together to form a paste. Apply to the face avoiding the area around the eyes. Leave the mask on until completely dry. Carefully wash it off using a warm, damp flannel. Give yourself a face mask once a week. Oily skin should also be treated with a vegetable facial oil.

Oily skin base oils

Suitable carrier oils include sweet almond, apricot kernel, peach kernel, evening primrose, borage seed and carrot oil.

Essential oils for oily skin

Bergamot, cedarwood, cypress, frankincense, geranium, juniper, lavender, lemon, palmarosa, petitgrain, rosemary, ylang ylang.

Suggested recipes for oily skin facial oils

Select any of the essential oils from the list above and add them to your chosen carrier oil(s). However, the following recipes are useful:

3 drops cedarwood 4 drops cypress 3 drops juniper	or	3 drops geranium 2 drops lemon 3 drops palmarosa 2 drops rosemary	or	2 drops bergamot 3 drops cypress 2 drops frankincense 3 drops petitgrain	diluted in 30 ml of carrier oil

Put all your ingredients into an amber-coloured bottle and shake well. Spots and blackheads may be treated individually with one drop of neat lavender or tea tree.

Diet

Oily skin is made worse by a diet rich in fatty foods and sugar. Eat lots of fruit and vegetables and plenty of fibre to avoid constipation which always makes oily skin worse. Avoid tea, coffee and cigarettes. Stress will also make skin break out.

Evening primrose oil and zinc may be helpful.

Normal skin care

You are fortunate if you have evenly balanced skin which is smooth, fine-pored, soft and supple, with no spots or blemishes. Children usually have this type of skin, whereas the rest of us have to work hard to achieve it.

There will always be times when this fine balance is disrupted – hormonal problems, illness and erratic diet can disturb the equilibrium.

Although normal skin needs no special extensive care it needs to be well looked after. Wash normal skin with a mild acid or pH-balanced soap daily in warm water. Apply a face mask once a week to ensure that the skin remains evenly balanced.

Face mask for normal skin
    2 tablespoons of clay/fuller's earth
    1 teaspoon honey
    1 teaspoon jojoba or avocado oil
    1 drop rose
    1 drop geranium or palmarosa

Mix the above ingredients to a thick paste. Apply to the face, avoiding the eye area. Relax.... Leave this mask on until it has dried. Then, gently wash it off with warm water. Use once weekly.

Normal skin should be treated with a facial oil at least once daily to stimulate and nourish the skin.

Normal skin base oils

Sweet almond, apricot kernel, jojoba, peach kernel, evening primrose oil and carrot oil are all suitable.

Essential oils for normal skin
Roman chamomile, frankincense, geranium, lavender, neroli, palmarosa, rose, rosewood.

Suggested recipes for normal skin facial oils

Select any of the essential oils from the list above and add them to your chosen carrier oil(s). You will find the following recipes useful:

4 drops geranium		3 drops frankincense	diluted in
3 drops rose	**or**	3 drops lavender	30 ml of
3 drops rosewood		4 drops palmarosa	carrier oil

A facial steambath is also beneficial occasionally. Follow the advice for oily skin but choose from the essential oils above.

Mature/ageing skin care

As we age, the skin deteriorates and wrinkles appear as the skin loses its elasticity. Mature skin needs moisture and oxygen.

Regular facial aromamassage can do a great deal to prevent and reduce wrinkling. After just a few treatments an improvement will be seen.

Massage stimulates the local circulation and, therefore, brings good supplies of oxygen to the inner living layers of the skin. Cell division slows down as we grow older and essential oils which stimulate cell growth (cytophylactic oils) are indicated. You can use aromatherapy oils to replace the moisture and treat dryness.

Anti-ageing base oils

Nourishing carrier oils such as avocado, jojoba, wheatgerm and peach and apricot kernel are excellent for mature skins.

Essential oils for anti-ageing

Roman chamomile, carrot seed, clary sage, frankincense, geranium, jasmine, lavender, neroli, palmarosa, rose, yarrow.

Suggested recipes for ageing skin facial oils

You may select any of the essential oils from the list above and add them to your chosen carrier oil(s). However, you may find the following recipes useful:

3 drops carrot seed		4 drops geranium	diluted in
3 drops frankincense	**or**	3 drops palmarosa	30 ml of
4 drops neroli		3 drops rose	carrier oil

If these oils are to be effective you must apply them to the face daily. Face packs are also invaluable for mature skins, removing waste products so that cells can be renewed more rapidly.

Face pack for ageing skin
The following recipe is recommended:

> 2 teaspoons ground almonds
> 1 teaspoon honey
> 2 teaspoons water (or rosewater/lavender water)

Mix the ingredients together and add one drop of essential oil of rose and 1 drop of frankincense. Apply to the face for ten to fifteen minutes. Rinse off gently.

Facial steambaths are also useful for mature skin to deep cleanse the pores and stimulate the circulation. Follow the instructions as for oily skin, using two drops of carrot seed, two drops of frankincense and two drops of neroli.

Diet
Adequate nutrition is essential for the skin. Try to consume only small amounts of alcohol, tea and coffee which help to create the wrinkles. Avoid sugary foods, and eat plenty of fruit and vegetables.

Exercise will help to increase the circulation and improve muscle tone. Avoid extremes of temperature.

Essential oils for skin problems

Acne
Acne occurs primarily during puberty but it can affect people well into their adult years. It is due to overactivity of the sebaceous (oil secreting) glands of the skin. Excessive sebum causes proliferation of bacteria, and the pores become blocked leading to blackheads and spots. It can lead to scarring.

Essential oils to clear the body toxins
Geranium, juniper, lemon, rosemary.

Essential oils to reduce and heal scarring
Carrot seed, frankincense, immortelle, lavender, mandarin, neroli.

Essential oils to promote the growth of new cells
Carrot seed, frankincense, lavender, neroli, palmarosa, patchouli, rosewood.

Essential oils to balance and reduce sebum
Clary sage, cypress, elemi, frankincense, geranium, lavender, lemongrass, yarrow, ylang ylang.

Essential oils as antiseptic and astringent
Bergamot, cedarwood, myrtle, yarrow.

Essential oils to soothe inflammation
Roman chamomile, yarrow.

Apply one drop of neat lavender or tea tree undiluted to individual spots. Wash the face with an unscented pH balanced or acid soap. A facial steam bath should be carried out twice a week. Facial oils should be applied daily.

Avoid refined, sweet and fatty foods, smoking, alcohol, tea, coffee and sugary drinks. Plenty of fruit and vegetables are essential as well as lots of water. Vitamin C, zinc and evening primrose oil will help. Exercise is also recommended.

Allergies (e.g. eczema)
Diet, pollutants and stress are all major causes of allergy rashes. It is important to try to identify the allergen – food, detergents, cosmetics or coarse clothing.

Useful essential oils
Roman chamomile, **melissa** and **yarrow** are three of my favourite oils which I use in the treatment of eczema. They certainly seem to reduce itching. Other oils include: **benzoin**, **geranium**, **lavender**, **frankincense**, **myrrh**, and **patchouli** (weeping eczema), **rose otto** and **sandalwood** (dry eczema).

Sometimes carrier oils can make eczema worse, so it is best to blend the essential oils with a non-perfumed organic base cream. The oils can also be applied in cold compresses. Baths are also highly effective.

Athlete's foot
This extremely itchy, infectious fungal condition thrives around and in between the toes. It loves warm and moist conditions.

Useful essential oils
Lavender, myrrh, lemongrass, patchouli and **tea tree**. Daily footbath using six drops of any of the above oils is recommended. Also dab neat lavender or tea tree on to the affected areas.

Broken capillaries

Weakness in the fine blood vessels can result in the appearance of fine, red veins usually on the cheeks. The capillaries are not really broken but are just weak and stretched. The capillary walls are supposed to be elastic, enlarging when the skin is hot and then shrinking back to their original size. If they lose their elasticity, they are prematurely dilated (enlarged) leading to a ruddy complexion.

Gentle facial massage can help to promote contraction of the blood vessels. Try the following formula over a period of months:

3 drops Roman chamomile   diluted in
3 drops parsley seed   30 ml of
4 drops rose   carrier oil

Cypress, frankincense, neroli and **patchouli** are also useful.

To enhance the treatment, avoid spicy foods, alcohol, smoking, caffeine and stress. Vitamin C is also beneficial.

Cellulite

Cellulite, sometimes referred to as 'orange peel skin', affects women almost exclusively, forming on the thighs, hips and buttocks and therefore it seems to be hormone related. It is characterised by lymphatic congestion, water retention, an increase in fatty tissue and often poor circulation.

Aromatherapy together with nutritional advice and exercise is quite a successful treatment for cellulite, if you persevere. The aim of the treatment is to stimulate the lymphatic system, balance the hormones and reduce the water retention. The following essential oils will be helpful:

Essential oils to reduce fluid
Cypress, fennel, grapefruit, juniper, lemon, lemongrass, rosemary, sandalwood, thyme.

Essential oils to stimulate the circulatory and detoxify the lymphatic systems
Basil, benzoin, black pepper, cedarwood, cypress, fennel, ginger, patchouli, rosemary, sage.

Essential oils to balance the hormones
Roman chamomile, clary sage, geranium, lavender, rose, sage.

Action plan for cellulite

1 Dry skin brushing daily. Brush in upward movements all over the body with a natural hair bristle brush, paying particular attention to the affected areas. This will detoxify and improve the circulation.

2 Bath at least once a day, choosing from the oils above or using one of the following formulae:

| 2 drops cypress
2 drops fennel
2 drops juniper | or | 2 drops black pepper
2 drops lemon
2 drops sage | or | 2 drops geranium
2 drops fennel
2 drops rose | diluted in 30 ml of carrier oil |

Follow the bath with a cold shower.

3 Massage the affected area twice daily – morning and evening – using the following formulae:

| 3 drops fennel
4 drops grapefruit
3 drops lemon | or | 3 drops cypress
3 drops geranium
4 drops juniper | diluted in 30 ml of carrier oil |

4 Pay attention to your diet. Eliminate tea, coffee and alcohol, drinking only spring water and herb teas – fennel tea is excellent. Eat plenty of fresh fruit and vegetables (raw if possible). Avoid sugar and refined carbohydrates as well as salty food. Avoid dairy foods from cows. Increase your vitamin C intake to at least 1 g daily.

5 Exercise daily for about twenty minutes – swimming and cycling are perfect.

6 Relaxation is vital as stress can affect the hormonal balance and elimination is less efficient.

Cold sores (herpes)

Cold sores are the result of lowered immunity, stress, extremes of temperature and excessively strong sunlight. They are caused by the herpes simplex virus. It is important to apply the essential oils at the first sign of an eruption. Dip a cotton bud into either of the following solutions and dab several times a day:

2 drops bergamot 2 drops lavender 1 drop lemon 3 drops tea tree	or	2 drops chamomile 1 drop eucalyptus 1 drop melissa 2 drops tea tree	diluted in 5 ml of vodka

Neat **lavender** or **tea tree** oil can also be used on the blisters. Take at least 1 g of vitamin C daily, 1000 mg of lysine and B complex. Eat plenty of fruit and vegetables and wholegrains.

Infectious skin conditions

Conditions such as chicken-pox, scabies and measles should never be massaged. Use six drops of any of the following oils in the bath: **bergamot, lavender, lemon, rosemary, tea tree.**

Psoriasis

This condition is characterised by the formulation of red patches which are covered by scaly skin, occurring mostly on the elbows, knees, palms of the hands, soles of the feet and on the head. Psoriasis is often inherited but may not appear until adulthood. The cause is unknown, although stress appears to be a major factor.

Psoriasis is a difficult condition to treat but it usually responds to aromatherapy.

Essential oils for psoriasis

Benzoin, bergamot, cajeput, Roman chamomile, lavender, niaouli and **yarrow.**

Any of the above oils may be blended with a carrier oil or mixed into a pure organic skin cream (see page 25 for details of creams).

Suggested recipes for psoriasis

Select any of the essential oils from the list above and add them to your chosen carrier oil(s). You may find the following recipes useful:

1 drop bergamot	diluted		2 drops benzoin	diluted in
3 drops Roman chamomile	in 30 ml carrier	or	4 drops Roman chamomile	30 g of pure organic skin cream
3 drops lavender			2 drops yarrow	
3 drops yarrow				

Avoid smoking and drinking alcohol and coffee. Fruit juices and water are beneficial. Fruit and vegetables (raw if possible) and simple wholefoods are recommended. Eat oily fish such as mackerel, sardines and tuna. Vitamins A, B complex, C, E, zinc and evening primrose oil may also be helpful. Moderate sun can also help psoriasis. Never wear unnatural fibres such as polyester or nylon next to the skin.

Hair

Just as our skin is a reflection of our inner health, so is our hair. The condition of our hair is, to a large extent, dependent on optimum health and nutrition. Hormonal changes, hereditary factors, stress, overexposure to ultraviolet rays, chemicals such as perms, dyes and hairsprays, pollutants and drugs will all affect the health of our hair. The health of our hair also depends upon the way that we treat it. It is vital that the hair is brushed thoroughly, preferably not with a nylon brush, to remove the old dead hair and stimulate natural growth. We have approximately 100,000 hairs on the scalp. Blonds have the most hair and the finest hair in comparison to redheads who have the least hair and the coarsest hair. Every day approximately eighty hairs are lost! My grandmother used to tell me to brush my hair 100 times a day and she was right; brushing massages the scalp, stimulates the circulation and removes old hair.

Essential oils are invaluable in hair care because they can influence and balance the sebaceous glands. The sebum which is secreted by these glands lubricates and protects the hair. If these glands are sluggish and underactive the hair will become dry and dehydrated. Conversely, if the sebaceous glands are overactive, the hair will become oily. Essential oils are beneficial to all types of hair for regulating the production of sebum.

Washing the hair

Many commercial shampoos contain chemical and synthetic substances which damage the scalp and the hair follicles. They attack the acid mantle of the scalp and wash away the hair's natural protective oils. Therefore, after each washing the hair should be rinsed with an acidic substance such as lemon juice or organic apple cider vinegar. This will wash out any residues of soap and will help to restore the acid equilibrium of the scalp.

You should avoid using the harsh detergent-based shampoos. Choose a mild natural shampoo which will be less likely to disturb the acid mantle of the scalp. You can even make your own shampoo using the following recipe:

> 100 g soap flakes (available from some health shops and pharmacies)
> 1 litre spring water

Simmer the spring water and add soap flakes, stirring until the flakes dissolve. Allow the mixture to cool and pour into a bottle or jar.

Add carrier oils and essential oils to this shampoo base, depending on your hair type.

Normal hair (healthy hair)

Normal hair is neither too dry nor too greasy, easy to comb, strong, self-renewing and shining. The following essential oils are useful to keep the hair healthy:

Essential oils for normal hair
Roman chamomile, carrot seed, geranium, lavender, lemon, parsley, rosemary, rosewood.

Roman chamomile and lemon are particularly effective for light hair. Carrot seed is good for ginger hair and rosemary and rosewood will enhance dark hair.

Suggested recipes for normal hair shampoo
Select any of the essential oils from the list above and add them to your shampoo base. You will find the following recipes useful:

Blonde hair	Dark hair	
8 drops Roman chamomile	4 drops carrot seed	mix together
	4 drops lemon	with 100 ml
3 drops carrot seed or	6 drops rosemary	shampoo
3 drops geranium	6 drops rosewood	base, and bottle
5 drops lemon		

Rinse for normal hair

> 1 cup of water
> 1 teaspoon of cider vinegar
> 3 drops lemon (blonde hair) or
> 3 drops rosemary (dark hair)

Deep, normal hair conditioning treatment and recipes

Once a week normal hair should be nourished with a deep conditioning hair treatment particularly if it is washed frequently or has been exposed to the sun, wind or chlorine in the swimming pool.

Dark hair	Blonde hair	
2 drops geranium ⎫ 2 drops rosemary ⎬ or 2 drops rosewood ⎭ 2 drops lemon	1 drop carrot seed ⎫ 3 drops Roman ⎬ chamomile ⎭	mixed with 2 tablespoons of jojoba oil/sweet almond oil/ peach kernel

Massage the oil thoroughly into the hair and then cover the head with a plastic shower cap. Leave the oil on the head for two hours or even overnight. Shampoo the hair as usual.

Dry hair

Dry hair is caused by the inactivity of the sebaceous glands. Aromatherapy treatment is directed towards stimulating the glands to restore the hair to its natural condition. Dry hair should always be protected from the sun, sea and swimming pools which can only aggravate the condition.

Essential oils for dry hair

Carrot seed, Roman chamomile, geranium, lavender, palmarosa, parsley, rosewood, sandalwood, ylang ylang.

Suggested recipes for dry hair shampoo

Select any of the essential oils from the list above and add them to the shampoo base.

You will find the following recipes useful:

4 drops carrot seed
4 drops lavender
6 drops palmarosa
6 drops ylang ylang

or

5 drops geranium
4 drops parsley
5 drops sandalwood
6 drops ylang ylang

blend well with 100 ml shampoo base and 1 teaspoon of jojoba or avocado or peach kernel carrier oil and bottle.

Rinse for dry hair
1 cup of water
1 teaspoon of cider vinegar
3 drops sandalwood **or**
3 drops ylang ylang

Blend the above ingredients well and add to the bowl of water you are using as your final rinse. Immerse your hair thoroughly.

Deep, dry hair conditioning treatment and recipe
It is essential to nourish dry hair which has often been damaged by bleach and other chemicals, as well as by the elements. Jojoba oil is particularly effective against dry, brittle hair and split ends. The following recipe is recommended and should be used at least once a week:

2 tablespoons jojoba oil
1 drop carrot seed
2 drops geranium
1 drop parsley
2 drops ylang ylang

Apply the above oil all over the scalp. Massage thoroughly and cover the hair with a plastic shower cap or polythene bag. Leave on for at least two hours or even overnight, then shampoo and rinse as usual.

Oily hair

Oily hair is caused by an overactivity of the sebaceous glands. This condition is exacerbated by shampooing too often with commercial shampoo, and the more you wash with these products the worse the condition becomes. If you use a mild shampoo then it is perfectly acceptable to wash it every day.

Essential oils for oily hair
Bergamot, cedarwood, clary sage, cypress, frankincense, juniper, lavender, lemon, rosemary, sage, thyme, yarrow.

Suggested recipe for oily hair shampoo
Select any of the essential oils from the list above and add them to the shampoo base. You will find the following recipe useful:

3 drops cedarwood ⎫
4 drops clary sage ⎪ blend well
4 drops cypress   ⎬ with 100 ml
7 drops lemon   ⎪ shampoo base,
2 drops yarrow   ⎭ and bottle

Rinse for oily hair
1 cup of water
2 teaspoon of cider vinegar (or lemon juice)
2 drops lemon
1 drop thyme

Blend the above ingredients well and add to your final rinse, ensuring that the whole scalp is effectively treated.

Hair tonic for oily hair
A hair tonic is particularly effective for oily hair. It should be massaged into the hair and left on overnight. This treatment should be carried out at least once a week and, if the condition is severe, two or three times.

2 cups of spring water (or boiled water)
2 tablespoons of apple cider vinegar/fresh lemon juice
2 drops bergamot
2 drops clary sage
3 drops cypress
2 drops lavender
1 drop thyme

Blend well and bottle. Rub into the scalp.

Deep, oily hair conditioning recipe and treatment
Oily hair needs to be conditioned about once a week.

2 tablespoons sweet almond oil
2 drops bergamot
2 drops cypress
2 drops lemon
2 drops yarrow

Blend the ingredients together and thoroughly massage the conditioner into the scalp. Cover the hair with a plastic shower cap or polythene bag. Leave for fifteen minutes. Then shampoo and rinse as usual.

Diet

Your hair reacts to the foods that you eat. Your diet provides you with all the necessary vitamins and minerals for a healthy head of hair, full of lustre. Avoid coffee, tea, alcohol, smoking, saturated fats and sugar. Eat plenty of fresh fruit and vegetables and unsaturated fatty acids.

Protect your hair as much as possible from strong sunlight, sea and chlorinated swimming pools. If you are going down to the beach for the day, why not apply a deep conditioning treatment. The warmth from the sun will enhance the effects of the treatment.

Try to relax as much as possible. Stress and tension can actually make you lose your hair.

Essential oils for other hair problems

Dandruff

Basil, carrot seed, Roman chamomile, cypress, eucalyptus, patchouli, peppermint, rosemary, sage and thyme are all beneficial for dandruff. Use them in your shampoo, rinses and hair oils. Always ensure that you rinse your hair thoroughly.

Hair loss

The following essential oils should be mixed into your hair products to stimulate hair growth: basil, Roman chamomile, cedarwood, clary sage, cypress, frankincense, geranium, ginger, lavender, peppermint, rosemary, sage, thyme and yarrow.

Head lice

As a mother of two children I have lots of experience in dealing with these. I have found the following essential oils to be effective: bergamot, eucalyptus, geranium, lavender, lemon, rosemary and tea tree.

Most children are unfortunately likely to pick up head lice at least once in their schooldays. Essential oils added to shampoos are a good preventive treatment. Also add one drop of rosemary and one drop of tea tree to the final rinse.

Lice treatment for children

2 tablespoons of carrier oil
1 drop lavender
1 drop lemon
1 drop rosemary
1 drop tea tree

Blend the ingredients together well, apply to the hair, cover with a polythene shower cap and leave overnight for maximum benefit. Comb through the hair thoroughly with a fine-toothed 'nit comb' available from chemists to remove lice and eggs. Shampoo and rinse as usual.

Never be embarrassed if your child has head lice. All children are vulnerable.

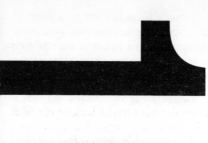
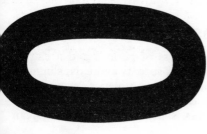

10

women's problems

In this chapter you will learn:
- the causes and effects of the most common 'women's problems'
- the orthodox treatment that is prescribed
- how aromatherapy is invaluable and why
- simple dietary and lifestyle changes to use alongside your aromatherapy treatment.

Women can be unfortunate enough to suffer from a host of problems. In this chapter I have covered premenstrual syndrome (PMS) and menopausal problems in detail as these are the two most common disorders that seem to present themselves at my clinic. I have covered the other 'women's problems' more briefly.

If your problem is severe or prolonged, please go to a gynaecologist to ensure that you do not have a serious medical condition.

Amenorrhoea (Absence of periods)

Amenorrhoea is the absence or loss of periods and it can be brought on by a number of factors, such as anorexia, slimming diets, strenuous physical training (e.g. athletics, gymnastics), disease of the ovaries or even coming off the contraceptive pill. Emotional upsets such as stress, shock and rapid changes can also result in amenorrhoea.

Aromatherapy treatment

If the problems are due to an emotional source, it should resolve itself in time. However, there are essential oils which encourage the menstrual cycle to re-establish itself again.

Useful oils include: **basil, carrot seed, Roman chamomile, clary sage, cypress, geranium, fennel, hyssop, juniper, marjoram, myrrh, parsley, peppermint, rose, rosemary, sage** and **thyme**.

Baths and sitz baths

Choose any combination of the above oils and put six drops into your daily bath or alternatively try a sitz bath. I recommend the following blend:

> 2 drops clary sage
> 2 drops cypress
> 2 drops marjoram
> 1 drop rose

Aromamassage

The following combination(s) of essential oils should be massaged into your abdomen and your low back daily for about a month.

2 drops cypress 2 drops fennel 2 drops juniper 1 drop marjoram	or	1 drop carrot seed 2 drops geranium 1 drop parsley seed 2 drops rose	diluted in 20 ml of carrier oil

It is beneficial to have a full body aromatherapy massage with either of the suggested blends on a weekly basis if stress has induced the amenorrhoea.

Contraindications
Do not use **fennel** excessively in case of epilepsy. **Sage, hyssop** and **thyme** also increase the blood pressure.

Bach Flower Remedies
The Remedy **Star of Bethlehem** is excellent for shock. Stressful situations also call for **Rescue Remedy**. Amenorrhoea caused by anorexia will require several remedies depending upon the individual – **Mimulus** is needed where there is a great fear (e.g. fear of getting fat), **Crab Apple** will help to cleanse away feelings of self-disgust and is for those who find food abhorrent, **Beech** is excellent for those who are self-critical, **Pine** is indicated for guilt and **Agrimony** for inner torture.

Diet
A healthy diet is essential to resolve problems of amenorrhoea. Once the menstrual difficulties have been attended to, the periods should return to normal.

Dysmenorrhoea (Painful periods)

Dysmenorrhoea or painful periods is a relatively common problem and the symptoms can vary from a slight ache to a violent cramping sensation that causes you to keel over and take to your bed. It is caused by cramp of the uterine muscles. There are two types of dysmenorrhoea – spasmodic cramping, a sharp pain often appearing on the first day of menstruation, and congestive cramping, a dull aching pain which usually starts prior to menstruation.

Aromatherapy treatment
Useful oils include: **angelica, Roman chamomile, cajeput, clary sage, cypress, fennel, ginger, jasmine, juniper, lavender, marjoram, melissa, peppermint, rose, rosemary** and **sage**.

Baths

You may experiment with different formulae to find the right combination for you, but the following may be useful:

2 drops Roman chamomile
2 drops clary sage
2 drops marjoram

Compresses

Aromatherapy compresses are one of the most effective ways of affording relief from menstrual pain. You may try any one of the oils from the list since they are all antispasmodic. Lavender and peppermint are an excellent combination (three drops each) as are Roman chamomile and marjoram. Clary sage and rose can also be used.

Aromamassage

This is particularly effective when performed on the abdomen or the low back area. Sometimes osteopathic treatment can bring relief from dysmenorrhoea. Massage the abdomen daily with one of the following blends:

2 drops clary sage 2 drops cypress 2 drops marjoram 1 drop rose	or	2 drops fennel 2 drops juniper 1 drop peppermint 1 drop sage	diluted in 20 ml of carrier oil

Contraindications

Avoid excessive use of **fennel** and **sage** in cases of epilepsy. Sage can increase the blood pressure.

Bach Flower Remedies

Rescue Remedy may be useful for pain relief. **Crab Apple** is recommended where there is congestion.

Diet

A healthy diet is essential with plenty of fruit and vegetables, cutting out sugar and refined foods. Useful supplements include evening primrose oil, calcium and magnesium.

Endometriosis

This is a condition whereby clumps of endometrial cells which normally line the uterus (the endometrium) appear and grow outside the uterus such as in the ovaries, Fallopian tubes, the bladder, intestines, lungs and elsewhere. It is still not clear how this problem develops.

Symptoms

Endometriosis affects at least over one million women in this country – I say at least as many cases of endometriosis remain undiagnosed for years. It is surprising that so little is written about it! Although the symptoms are variable they include painful periods, pain on ovulation and intercourse, heavy bleeding, erratic bleeding, pain when emptying the bowels or passing water, infertility, nausea, anxiety and depression. The pain can be absolutely excruciating with the sufferer rolling around the floor in agony.

Treatment

Orthodox treatment

Drugs such as Danozol, a testosterone drug which has many unpleasant side effects are prescribed. A laparoscopy may be performed in order to examine the abdomen. Sometimes surgery is necessary.

Aromatherapy treatment

Aromatherapy is helpful in some cases for relieving the pain and to relax the sufferer. Stress undoubtedly makes the pain much worse.

Useful oils include: **bergamot, Roman chamomile, cypress, geranium, lavender, peppermint, rose, sage** and **yarrow**.

Sitz baths

Although aromatherapy baths are relaxing, hot and cold sitz baths are particularly recommended for endometriosis. The aim of this treatment is to encourage the blood vessels to contract and to dilate. You will need two washing-up bowls for this method (baby baths are ideal, too). Fill up one bowl with hot water and one with cold water. Sit in the hot sitz bath for ten minutes and then in the cold sitz bath for five minutes. Repeat this procedure two or three times (you may need to add some more hot water to the hot bath).

The following blend should be added to the hot bath only:

1 drop Roman chamomile
1 drop clary sage
2 drops cypress
2 drops geranium
1 drop rose

The hot and cold sitz baths should be carried out daily. If you find this method impossible then add the blend to your bath instead.

Aromamassage
Massage the abdomen and the low back area every day using one of the following formulae:

| 2 drops Roman chamomile 3 drops cypress 2 drops yarrow | **or** | 2 drops clary sage 3 drops geranium 1 drop rose | diluted in 20 ml of carrier oil |

In order to get results the aromatherapy baths and daily massages should be carried out for several months. Do persevere!

Compresses
Alternate hot or cold compresses may be used to provide pain relief. **Peppermint, clary sage** and **lavender** are probably the most effective essential oils. Into a small bowl of water put two drops of clary sage, two drops of lavender, and two drops of peppermint. Soak up the solution on to your flannel, squeeze it out and place it on to the abdomen or lower back area – wherever the pain is most severe.

A peppermint compress will also be useful in cases of nausea.

Contraindications
Do not use **fennel** or **sage** excessively in cases of epilepsy. Sage can raise the blood pressure. Avoid **peppermint** if taking homoeopathic medication.

Bach Flower Remedies
To ease the physical and emotional tension it is well worth trying some **Rescue Remedy**.

Diet

A healthy diet, exercise and relaxation should also be followed by those with endometriosis. Avoid stress as much as possible. Evening primrose oil can help to relieve the pain and cramping.

Menopause

The menopause usually occurs somewhere between the ages of forty-five to fifty-five and means the end of the monthly menstruation cycle. Although some women stop menstruating abruptly, most women experience an erratic cycle for several years prior to the cessation of menstruating. It is a gradual process. Nowadays many people regard the menopause as an illness when in fact it is a normal state of a woman's development.

Symptoms

The most commonly experienced symptoms include hot flushes, heavy night sweating, irregular periods with scanty or heavy bleeding (flooding), dizziness and fainting, irritability, insomnia, depression, memory loss, headaches, constipation and weight gain, cold hands and feet, and increased or reduced libido. Blood pressure also rises after the menopause, vaginal dryness can occur and some women experience hair loss.

It is interesting that women who are stressed or who lead a physically and sexually inactive life have far more problems in the menopause.

Treatment

Orthodox treatment

Consists of hormone replacement therapy (HRT). Although this treatment increases bone density – but **only** when you are taking it – it does have side effects. It can lead to hypertension, weight gain and has been linked with an increased risk of cancer of the breast and uterus. More research is needed to investigate possible side-effects.

Aromatherapy treatment

My advice is to try essential oils, which can have a remarkable effect on the regulation of hormones. Aromatherapy coupled with the right diet and an exercise programme can offer an alternative to HRT. The menopause should be approached in a positive way instead of with feelings of dread.

Although all women will have a different experience of the menopause I have found the following essential oils to be helpful with my patients: **bergamot, Roman chamomile, clary sage, cypress, fennel, frankincense, geranium, jasmine, juniper, lavender, lemon, melissa, neroli, peppermint, rose, rosemary, sage, sandalwood, violet leaf, yarrow** and **ylang ylang**.

On an emotional level there are many essential oils which can help to alleviate the depression and irritability of the menopause. Bergamot is a wonderfully uplifting oil as is clary sage which can induce a sense of well-being. Chamomile is invaluable for relieving the nervous tension associated with the menopause. Cypress not only relieves irritability and stress but is also invaluable for times of change, easing the transition.

The menopause, of course, is often referred to as 'the change'. Frankincense will enable a woman to move on and enjoy the freedom and exhilaration that the menopause can offer. Geranium is sedative yet uplifting and is also a balancer of the hormones and the skin. The exquisite aromas of jasmine, neroli and rose cannot fail to lift depression and induce optimism, euphoria and confidence. Violet leaf relieves anger and irritability.

On a physical level there are essential oils which will deal with the uncomfortable and embarrassing hot flushes caused by the irregular function of the blood vessels as they contract and dilate. Peppermint, cypress, clary sage, geranium, lemon, sage and violet leaf are all useful for these symptoms. To counteract fluid retention, bloating and constipation, cypress, fennel, geranium, juniper, lemon, rosemary and sage may be applied. Insomnia may be relieved by putting a few drops of clary sage, chamomile, lavender or ylang ylang on your pillow. Chamomile, geranium, rose and yarrow are often employed to regulate the menstrual cycle. To help with circulation geranium, peppermint and rosemary are beneficial.

Baths

Daily aromatherapy baths are an enormous help as you go through the menopause. Try some of the following blends or choose from my list.

Nerve balancing formulae:

2 drops Roman chamomile		2 drops clary sage	
3 drops cypress	or	2 drops frankincense	
2 drops rose		2 drops lavender	

Hot flushes formula:

2 drops cypress
2 drops peppermint
2 drops sage

Bloated/constipation formula:

2 drops fennel
2 drops rosemary
2 drops sage

Aromamassage

Aromamassage is an excellent way of pampering and nurturing a woman as she goes through 'the change'. It increases self-esteem and can make her feel positive, confident and feminine. It is excellent for minimising the physical problems, too. Try the following formulae:

Uplifting formulae:

2 drops bergamot
1 drop Roman chamomile
2 drops cypress
2 drops rose

or

2 drops frankincense
2 drops geranium
1 drop jasmine
1 drop melissa

diluted in
20 ml of
carrier oil

Hot flushes/sweating formula:

2 drops cypress
2 drops lemon
2 drops peppermint
2 drops sage

diluted in
20 ml of
carrier oil

Cold hands and feet formula:

1 drop black pepper
2 drops mandarin
2 drops geranium
2 drops rosemary

diluted in
20 ml of
carrier oil

For emergencies you may like to keep a bottle of essential oil of peppermint in your handbag and inhale to help a hot flush.

Fluid retention/bloatedness formula:

2 drops cypress
2 drops mandarin
2 drops juniper
1 drop rosemary

diluted in
20 ml of
carrier oil

If you find that you are suffering from confusion and a poor memory, try inhaling a few drops of rosemary from a tissue every day. For formulae for vaginal dryness, and loss of libido please refer to Chapter 12. For hair loss and skin problems refer to Chapter 09. For poor circulation and high blood pressure refer to Chapter 06.

Contraindications

Avoid excessive use of **fennel** and **sage** if you are epileptic. Sage can raise the blood pressure. Do not apply **bergamot** and **lemon** before sunbathing. Avoid **peppermint** when taking homoeopathic medications.

Bach Flower Remedies

Walnut is the most important Remedy during the menopause as it assists 'change'. **Larch** is excellent for restoring confidence. For feelings of hopelessness and despair try **Gorse**. For mood swings and indecision **Scleranthus** can be very helpful. Use **Impatiens** for irritability and **Willow** for resentment. **Olive** is essential for fatigue and tiredness.

Diet

Diet is important as women go through the menopause if osteoporosis is to be prevented. Calcium-rich foods should be increased to maintain strong and healthy bones. These include fish such as sardines where the bones are eaten, sunflower, pumpkin and sesame seeds, nuts and dairy foods if they can be tolerated. Since calcium requires vitamin D in order to be absorbed it is vital to go out into the sunshine. Exercise – especially skipping or jumping on the spot – can increase your bone density.

As calorie needs decline with the onset of the menopause you must eat less. Avoid salt and refined sugar. Reduce tea, coffee and alcohol. Increase your intake of fruit, vegetables and fibre. Try vitamin C (1 g daily) and evening primrose oil for the hot flushes. Take an iron supplement to counteract blood loss if there is 'flooding' and vitamin B-complex, zinc, vitamin C, calcium, and magnesium for stress. Calcium and magnesium are also vital for preventing the loss of bone.

Relaxation is important – aromatherapy baths and massage are ideal. Remember also to think positively.

Menorrhagia (Heavy bleeding)

Menorrhagia is profuse bleeding often with clotting. Abnormally heavy bleeding can occur at any time during a woman's life, but it is particularly common around the time of the menopause. Naturally, profuse bleeding or bleeding between periods should always be diagnosed by the doctor to ensure that there is no serious medical condition.

Aromatherapy treatment

Once the menorrhagia has been checked out, aromatherapy treatment can begin with the aim of regulating the periods.

Useful oils include: **Roman chamomile, cypress, frankincense, geranium, juniper, lemon, rose** and **yarrow**.

Baths/sitz baths

Any of the essential oils above may be added to your bath or in a sitz bath.

3 drops geranium 3 drops lemon	or	2 drops cypress 2 drops frankincense 2 drops yarrow	or	3 drops juniper 3 drops lemon use this formula when the womb needs cleansing

Aromamassage

The abdomen and lower back can be massaged gently every day with one of the following blends:

2 drops Roman chamomile 2 drops frankincense 2 drops geranium 1 drop yarrow	or	2 drops cypress 2 drops lemon 2 drops rose	diluted in 20 ml of carrier oil

Contraindications

Avoid **lemon** prior to sunbathing.

Bach Flower Remedies

Crab Apple is indicated if cleansing is required. Use **Rescue Remedy** to provide pain relief.

Diet

A healthy diet is essential. It should be remembered that heavy periods can result in iron deficiency (anaemia). Please refer to pages 97–9 for details on this condition. Kelp can correct profuse bleeding caused by a thyroid deficiency.

Premenstrual syndrome (PMS)

The above term is used to describe the wide range of symptoms which affect women in the second half of the menstrual cycle. Women can be affected anything from three days to two weeks prior to menstruation.

Symptoms

Over 150 symptoms have been attributed to PMS, although most women thankfully will suffer from just a few of them. The most common physical and psychological symptoms include:

- anxiety, irritability and mood swings
- bloating of the abdomen
- breast tenderness
- fatigue, fainting and dizziness
- feelings of aggression, violence and suicide
- fluid retention
- headaches and migraine
- increased appetite and cravings for sweet things
- lack of concentration, confusion, clumsiness and forgetfulness
- skin problems
- weight gain

In Western societies there has been a vast increase in PMS.

Treatment

Orthodox treatment
May involve taking the contraceptive pill and drugs to relieve anxiety. Some doctors now recommend supplements such as evening primrose oil.

Aromatherapy treatment

Aromatherapy is invaluable and it has helped enormous numbers of sufferers to overcome this distressing condition. When selecting your essential oils, both the physical and emotional problems should be addressed. For maximum benefit, it is vital that they are used alongside a nutritional programme.

Every woman has a different experience of PMS and, therefore, it is impossible to provide one solution for this hormonal imbalance. However, the following essential oils have been found to be successful: **benzoin, bergamot, carrot seed, cedarwood, Roman chamomile, clary sage, cypress, fennel, frankincense, geranium, grapefruit, jasmine, juniper, lemon, melissa, neroli, parsley, rose, rosemary, sage, sandalwood** and **ylang ylang.**

On an emotional level there are many essential oils that can help to reduce anxiety and uplift depression. Benzoin is renowned for its warming effects on the emotions and bergamot is effective for alleviating depression. Cedarwood calms and soothes nervous states and carrot seed relieves tension and exhaustion. Roman chamomile eases anger, irritability, and balances mood swings. Clary sage is a wonderful euphoric-sedative oil which can calm an overactive mind inducing feelings of optimism. Cypress is a comforting oil ideal for relieving states of anger and irritability. Frankincense instils feelings of calmness and serenity and geranium balances the nervous system. Grapefruit is refreshing and reviving for a listless, apathetic state of mind. Jasmine is a marvellous oil for uplifting depression encouraging positive thoughts and actions. Melissa is soothing and calming, dispelling melancholy and neroli is invaluable for bringing peace and tranquillity to an agitated mind. Palmarosa helps to raise a low self-esteem and parsley soothes and calms aggression. Rose exerts a profound effect on the emotions and is recommended for particularly difficult cases! Sandalwood and ylang ylang are deeply relaxing releasing anger and tension.

On a physical level cypress, fennel, geranium, juniper, lemon, rosemary and sage are excellent oils to help to minimise or completely eradicate fluid retention. They are all excellent detoxifiers.

Breast tenderness can be soothed by oils such as Roman chamomile, cypress, geranium and rose.

Fennel is one of the most effective oils for helping to balance the appetite and will, therefore, help to reduce the cravings for cakes, chocolate and sweets which is so characteristic of PMS. It will also prevent weight gain. Headaches may be calmed and soothed with compresses of Roman chamomile, peppermint and lavender.

Baths

Aromatherapy baths should be taken on a daily basis. The following blends may be helpful but, as usual, I urge you to select your oils from the list until you find a combination which absolutely suits you.

Fluid retention formulae:

2 drops cypress
1 drop fennel
2 drops juniper
1 drop sage
} or {
2 drops geranium
2 drops lemon
2 drops rosemary
}

Anger/irritability formulae:

2 drops Roman chamomile
2 drops geranium
2 drops ylang ylang
} or {
2 drops bergamot
3 drops palmarosa
1 drop parsley
}

Depression formulae:

2 drops bergamot
3 drops clary sage
1 drop rose
} or {
2 drops cedarwood
2 drops jasmine
2 drops melissa
}

Fatigue formulae:

2 drops carrot seed
2 drops grapefruit
2 drops lemon
} or {
3 drops lemon
2 drops rosemary
1 drop sage
}

Aromamassage

Aromamassage, especially lymphatic drainage techniques, can assist enormously with fluid retention. A full body massage should be carried out a day or two prior to the onset of the fluid retention. Self-massage of the affected areas is also highly recommended.

Massage is also the best method of reducing the psychological symptoms. It gives the woman some time to relax and unwind, to get things into proportion once again. The following blends are useful:

Fluid retention formula:

2 drops cypress ⎫ diluted
2 drops geranium ⎬ in
2 drops juniper ⎬ 20 ml of
1 drop rosemary ⎭ carrier oil

Anxiety/mood swing formulae:

3 drops Roman ⎫   2 drops bergamot ⎫ diluted in
   chamomile ⎬   2 drops clary sage ⎬ 20 ml of
1 drop palmarosa ⎬ or   2 drops geranium ⎬ carrier
2 drops rose ⎭   1 drop rose ⎭ oil

A combination of massage and daily baths is the best way to combat PMS. You can inhale essential oils from a handkerchief which can have a profound effect on the nervous system, or the oils may be placed into a clay burner.

Contraindications

Avoid **fennel** and **sage** excessively in epilepsy. **Bergamot, grapefruit** and **lemon** should not be applied prior to sunbathing. Sage raises the blood pressure.

Bach Flower Remedies

Walnut is an excellent remedy to use throughout the menstrual cycle as it is indicated for adjustments and change and this is what the menstrual cycle is. **Impatiens** should be used for anger, irritability and impatience which are all major symptoms of PMS. **Mustard** is indicated for depression which is also a common feature. **Cherry Plum** is the Remedy for suicidal tendencies and a fear of losing control. **Crab Apple** is invaluable for those feelings of self-disgust and ugliness which often accompany the bloatedness, spots and blemishes which may occur. **Willow** will help feelings of self-pity which women can experience premenstrually. Finally **Hornbeam** is beneficial for fatigue and lethargy, encouraging an optimistic and enthusiastic outlook.

Diet

Since the increase in the number of PMS sufferers has risen partly due to the changes in dietary habits which have occurred, attention to diet is a crucial part of any PMS programme. Dr Guy Abraham, PMS pioneer, claims that 90 per cent of women will respond to a nutritional programme.

Dietary recommendations for PMS:

1 Reduce salt consumption which leads to fluid retention and weight gain
2 Reduce the consumption of refined sugar which leads to psychological symptoms
3 Reduce drinks which contain caffeine (coffee, tea, cola) and alcohol which aggravate psychological symptoms
4 Reduce fats and protein
5 Increase your fibre intake by eating plenty of green, leafy vegetables, fruits and legumes to aid the elimination of toxins.

Supplements which PMS sufferers have found to be useful include evening primrose oil, B vitamins (especially B6), magnesium and vitamin C.

It is also essential to reduce stress – aromatherapy, of course, is a wonderful way to relax. Gentle exercise such as yoga, swimming or walking can also decrease tension, improve circulation and prevent fluid retention.

Oils for other problems

The following essential oils may be applied, using any of the methods outlined in Chapter 03. Sitz baths, compresses and gentle massage of the abdomen and low back are particularly recommended for the treatment of women's problems.

Cystitis
Angelica, bergamot, cajeput, cedarwood, eucalyptus, frankincense, garlic, juniper, lavender, myrtle, niaouli, sandalwood, tea tree and thyme.

Herpes
Bergamot, eucalyptus, geranium, immortelle, garlic, lavender, lemon and niaouli.

Infertility
Basil, carrot seed, clary sage, geranium, jasmine, melissa and rose.

Leucorrhea (white/yellow vaginal discharge)
Benzoin, bergamot, cedarwood, eucalyptus, hyssop, juniper, lavender, myrrh, myrtle, rose, rosemary, sage, sandalwood and thyme.

Thrush (candida)
Bergamot, eucalyptus, frankincense, lavender, lemon, myrrh, patchouli, rosemary, rosewood, sage, tea tree and thyme.

Vaginitis (vaginal inflammation)
German chamomile, clary sage, lavender, sandalwood, tea tree and thyme.

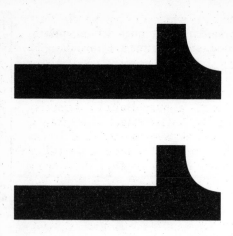

1

pregnancy, childbirth, babies and children

In this chapter you will learn:
- how aromatherapy may be used to treat a wide range of conditions throughout pregnancy
- how essential oils can help new mothers during and after childbirth
- how babies and children can benefit from aromatherapy.

Aromatherapy may be used successfully throughout the forty weeks of pregnancy to treat a wide range of conditions. Although no one can guarantee a healthy, normal baby, the risks can be substantially reduced if the mother takes good care of herself and follows a healthy diet (see page 178 for dietary advice) and maintains a balanced state of mind (see page 177 for Bach Flower Remedies). There is a great deal of controversy about which oils to avoid in the various stages of pregnancy, particularly during the first trimester. But provided essential oils are used *correctly* and in the *appropriate* dilutions, the risk is slight. In my own practice I have been privileged to treat many pregnant women with excellent results and *no* harmful side effects. Indeed on both occasions when I was pregnant I was fortunate to be able to practise aromatherapy until the deliveries. Every week, on average, I was probably using about twenty to thirty different blends of essential oils on my patients. Both my pregnancies were problem-free with easy births without orthodox analgesia and two extremely healthy babies. I am certain that I could not have achieved this without my precious essential oils.

Although you should be aware of the potential hazards of some essential oils, it is vital to keep it all in perspective. Instead of giving you a long list of so-called hazardous oils – some of which are referred to with no proof – I recommend that you use the oils which I have indicated for each condition. Naturally if symptoms are severe or persist then the advice of a doctor should *always* be sought.

Common ailments in pregnancy

Backache

Backache can become so severe that the mother can be incapacitated. Essential oils are marvellous for treating backache and they can be added to the bath, blended into a back-rub or used in compresses.

Essential oils for backache
Roman chamomile, black pepper, frankincense, geranium, ginger, lavender, sweet marjoram.

Add six drops of any of the above oils to a warm bath and relax or make a compress. For a back massage the following combinations may be useful:

$$\left.\begin{array}{l}\text{2 drops Roman} \\ \quad\text{chamomile} \\ \text{1 drop geranium} \\ \text{1 drop lavender}\end{array}\right\} \text{or} \left.\begin{array}{l}\text{1 drop frankincense} \\ \text{1 drop ginger} \\ \text{1 drop rose}\end{array}\right\} \begin{array}{l}\text{diluted} \\ \text{in 10 ml} \\ \text{of carrier} \\ \text{oil}\end{array}$$

Constipation

It is vital for the pregnant woman to eat lots of 'natural foods' with plenty of fruit, vegetables and fibre. Also drink lots of water. Pregnancy is *not* the time to take chemical laxatives, which could be dangerous. Natural laxatives such as prunes are recommended and work excellently in combination with aromatherapy to ensure a regular bowel action.

Essential oils for constipation
Black pepper, Roman chamomile, lavender, lemon, patchouli, rose and sweet marjoram.

These oils may be used in a bath up to a maximum of six drops in total. The best method is to make up a massage blend and rub it into the abdomen in a clockwise direction (see *Teach Yourself Massage* for a full description of abdominal massage).

Aromatic formulae for constipation

$$\left.\begin{array}{l}\text{2 drops black pepper} \\ \text{1 drop lavender} \\ \text{1 drop sweet} \\ \quad\text{marjoram}\end{array}\right\} \text{or} \left.\begin{array}{l}\text{2 drops Roman} \\ \quad\text{chamomile} \\ \text{1 drop patchouli} \\ \text{1 drop rose}\end{array}\right\} \begin{array}{l}\text{diluted} \\ \text{in 10 ml} \\ \text{of carrier} \\ \text{oil}\end{array}$$

Cramp

Cramps in the legs appear to be more prevalent during the last months of the pregnancy and are often worse during the night. One possible cause may be a lack of calcium.

Essential oils for cramps
Roman chamomile, cypress, frankincense, geranium, lavender, sweet marjoram and rosemary.

These oils may be used successfully in a footbath, or the legs can be *gently* massaged upwards from the ankle to the thigh.

Footbath for leg cramps

2 drops cypress
1 drop frankincense
1 drop geranium
2 drops lavender

Aromatic formulae for leg cramps

2 drops Roman chamomile
2 drops cypress
2 drops lavender

or

2 drops Roman chamomile
2 drops geranium
2 drops sweet marjoram

diluted in 10 ml of carrier oil

Fatigue

Extreme tiredness can be a problem in pregnancy, especially if the woman has other children to care for.

Essential oils for fatigue

Bergamot, geranium, grapefruit, lavender, lemon, lemongrass, lime, mandarin, neroli and **rosemary**.

For a 'quick fix' burst of energy the best method is inhalation. Sprinkle a couple of drops of the above oils – the citrus oils are particularly effective – on to a tissue and inhale deeply.

Alternatively, add six drops of any of the recommended oils to a bath or footbath or treat yourself to a massage using one of the following blends:

2 drops bergamot
2 drops geranium
2 drops lemon

or

2 drops grapefruit
2 drops lime
2 drops neroli

diluted in 10 ml of carrier oil

Morning sickness

Although nausea is commonly experienced during the early stages, some women are unlucky enough to be subject to it right through pregnancy.

Essential oils for nausea

Ginger, lavender, lemon, mandarin, melissa, peppermint, petitgrain, rosewood.

The best method of using essential oils for morning sickness is by inhalation. Simply sprinkle two to three drops of any of the recommended oils on to a tissue, handkerchief or cotton wool ball and inhale deeply. You may also add them to your morning bath. A particularly lovely combination is two drops of ginger, two drops of mandarin, and two drops of petitgrain. A few sips of apple or orange juice prior to rising can prevent the excessive drop in blood sugar which accompanies nausea. A piece of dry toast or a biscuit before getting up can also be effective.

Stretch marks

In order to prevent unsightly stretch marks, massage the abdomen twice daily in a clockwise direction. This has worked for me and all my patients. Massage of the abdomen is also a wonderful way to establish contact and form a strong bond with your baby.

Essential oils for preventing stretch marks

Carrot seed, Roman chamomile, frankincense, geranium, lavender, lemon, mandarin, neroli and rose.

As well as massaging the abdomen, you should also treat other areas which are susceptible to stretch marks – thighs, buttocks, breasts and upper chest.

Aromatic formula for stretch marks

1 drop carrot seed	diluted in
2 drops frankincense	30 ml
2 drops lavender	of
2 drops mandarin	carrier
2 drops neroli	oil
1 drop rose	

Make up the above blend, shake well and store it in an amber-coloured glass bottle. Add a little wheatgerm oil to whichever carrier oil(s) you have selected.

Varicose veins

To prevent the arrival of varicose veins caused by the extra pressure on the legs, pregnant women should ideally rest with their legs raised for at least half an hour a day. If you can manage to raise them several times a day for five to ten minutes this will also help considerably.

Essential oils for varicose veins

Cypress, geranium, lavender, lemon and sandalwood.

Gentle massage of the legs twice a day is also an excellent preventive treatment.

Aromatic formula for varicose veins

1 drop cypress ⎫ diluted
1 drop geranium ⎪ in 10 ml
1 drop lemon ⎬ of carrier
1 drop sandalwood ⎭ oil

Footbaths are also quite effective. Try two drops each of cypress, geranium and lemon in a bowl of hand hot water.

Bach Flower Remedies in pregnancy

During pregnancy women experience a variety of emotional ups and downs as well as the physical conditions described above. The Bach Flower Remedies are an excellent way of maintaining balance throughout the nine months of pregnancy. They are harmless and cause no side effects. **Walnut** is essential for coping with the enormous physical and emotional changes that take place so quickly in pregnancy.

Star of Bethlehem is for counteracting the shock. Even when pregnancies are planned it still comes as a big shock when it actually happens. **Mimulus** is to alleviate the fears that the mother may be harbouring. Will the baby be normal? Can I cope with the pain? Will there be any complications? **Olive** is to combat fatigue and tiredness which is so often experienced. **Red Chestnut** is for overconcern for the baby's welfare. I have treated some pregnant women who have not wanted to have a bath in case it damages the baby. **Impatiens** is particularly useful towards the end of pregnancy when the end is in sight. Women understandably feel impatient and frustrated that the baby is not here, particularly when it is overdue. **Rescue Remedy** is ideal for the stages of labour when women can panic and lose control. If the mind is not relaxed then the contractions will be more painful. **Mustard** is the classic remedy for post-natal depression which descends out of the blue for no apparent reason. Star of Bethlehem should be taken if the birth was traumatic as well as Walnut to make the transition easier.

Diet in pregnancy

To give your baby the best possible start I recommend the following guidelines:

- Eat plenty of fresh fruit and vegetables, especially dark green, leafy vegetables, wholegrains and an adequate amount of protein;
- Avoid refined carbohydrates (cakes, biscuits, sweets), processed foods, foods with artificial additives and excessive tea and coffee;
- Take a vitamin and mineral supplement and folic acid, if possible, prior to conception;
- Avoid excessive vitamin A which can cause congenital malformations. In the United Kingdom the Department of Health advises women not to eat liver due to its high vitamin A content;
- Avoid alcohol which has been associated with abnormalities;
- Stop smoking which has been associated with a low birth weight;
- Avoid drugs. Check out all your medications whether prescribed by your doctor or bought over the counter;
- Avoid refined soft cheeses (e.g. camembert), paté, uncooked eggs (and mayonnaise), raw or uncooked meats and unpasteurised milk;
- Wash your hands after coming into contact with animals.

Oils for other pregnancy problems

Haemorrhoids
Cypress, frankincense, geranium, lavender, myrrh and sandalwood. Best method: sitz bath

Heartburn
Bergamot, coriander, dill, ginger, mandarin, peppermint, spearmint and sandalwood. Best method: massage of abdomen

Hypertension (high blood pressure)
Roman chamomile, lavender, sandalwood and ylang ylang. Best method: inhalation/bath/massage

Insomnia
Roman chamomile, lavender, mandarin, marjoram (sweet), neroli, sandalwood and ylang ylang. Best method: inhalation/bath/ massage

Mood swings/depression
Bergamot, clary sage, cedarwood, cypress, geranium, mandarin, neroli, rose and rosewood. Best method: inhalation/bath/massage

Oedema
Cypress, geranium, lemon and mandarin. Best method: massage

Urinary tract infections
Bergamot, Roman chamomile, juniper, sandalwood and tea tree. Best method: sitz bath

Vaginal infections
Bergamot, lavender, myrrh and tea tree. Best method: sitz bath

Childbirth

Essential oils are increasing in popularity with midwives, and some hospitals even have a stock of their own. Giving birth is extremely hard work but it is a wonderful, rewarding experience. Essential oils can stimulate the uterus to contract, facilitating the birth, and enable the mother to relax, thus affording pain relief.

Essential oils for labour

Bergamot, clary sage, frankincense, geranium, jasmine, lavender, mandarin, marjoram, neroli, palmarosa, peppermint, petitgrain, rose otto, and ylang ylang.

Aromatic formulae for labour

3 drops clary sage 2 drops mandarin 1 drop rose 2 drops ylang ylang }	or	2 drops frankincense 2 drops lavender 2 drops neroli 2 drops palmarosa }	diluted in 10 ml of carrier oil

The oils may be massaged into the back with the mother in a side-lying position or on all fours (see *Teach Yourself Massage* for special techniques), or the mother's feet can be massaged. The oils may also be inhaled on a tissue or cotton-wool ball as an alternative to gas and air or used in a diffuser or vaporiser. Compresses are also excellent for pain relief.

Post-natal care

Essential oils are invaluable after childbirth not only for physical problems but also to prevent or banish stress, anxiety and post-natal depression.

Breastfeeding

Breast milk is, of course, the best possible start for your baby, providing antibodies to disease and reducing the risk of allergies. However, it is not always easy to breastfeed. Essential oils can usually provide the answer.

To promote the milk supply

Fennel, clary sage, jasmine and **lemongrass** can all help to promote lactation – an old-fashioned remedy is to chew fennel seeds. Drink fennel tea daily and massage the breasts three times a day after feeding time (not the nipples). Massage almond oil or wheatgerm oil into the nipples to prevent cracking. Ensure that you wash the breasts prior to a feed.

Aromatic formula for increasing milk supply

3 drops fennel	diluted in
2 drops lemongrass	20 ml of
1 drop clary sage	carrier oil

I can assure you that essential oils can promote the milk supply. I breastfed my daughter until she was fifteen months old and my son until he was two years old. If you do have no desire to breastfeed or perhaps wish to give up, the following oils will help to stop lactation: **cypress, geranium, lavender, peppermint** and **sage**. Peppermint and sage are particularly useful. Try this blend:

Aromatic formula for decreasing milk supply

2 drops cypress	diluted in
3 drops peppermint	20 ml of
2 drops sage	carrier oil

Peppermint, sage and geranium compresses are also good.

Mastitis

This is a common, painful disorder of the breasts. A compress with two drops of **Roman chamomile**, one drop of **geranium**, one drop of **lavender** and one drop of **peppermint** will help to cool down the inflammation.

Healing the perineum

The perineum can become badly damaged during the birth process, particularly if you have torn badly or have had a forceps delivery. Aromatherapy sitz baths can increase the rate of healing, decrease the pain and fight off any infections. Compresses are also highly recommended.

Aromatic sitz bath for the perineum

2 drops Roman
  chamomile
2 drops lavender   } or { 2 drops cypress
2 drops tea tree   1 drop frankincense
                              1 drop myrrh
                              2 drops tea tree

If you have been unfortunate enough to have a Caesarean section, baths and compresses with three drops of **lavender** and three drops of **tea tree** will help the healing process.

Post-natal depression

Although a few women suffer no emotional imbalance at all, the majority suffer from the 'baby blues' a few days after the birth. There are many essential oils to strengthen the nervous system and uplift the despondency and despair.

Essential oils for the 'baby blues'

Bergamot, clary sage, frankincense, geranium, grapefruit, jasmine, mandarin, melissa, neroli and **rose.**

Choose one oil or a combination from the list above using a maximum of six drops in the bath. The new mother should also take some time out each week to indulge herself in an aromatherapy massage.

Aromatherapy for babies

Babies love essential oils, particularly if their mother has used them throughout her pregnancy, and they respond so rapidly to them. The use of essential oils helps to boost the immune system and if the body does become ill, the recovery will be much more speedy and the baby will experience far less discomfort.

Massage is a powerful and wonderful way for the parents to bond with their baby – I have described a detailed massage routine in *Teach Yourself Massage*.

Essential oils are used in low dilutions for aromamassage and baths. Babies should *never* be given essential oils internally. For babies up to the age of twelve months, the appropriate dilutions are:

Babies (0–2 months)   1 drop per 15 ml carrier oil in a massage; 1 drop in the bath.
Babies (2–12 months)   1 drop per 10 ml carrier oil in a massage; 1 drop in the bath.

Colic

Colic is a distressing condition for both the baby and the parents. The baby continues to cry even when picked up, which makes the parents feel helpless. However, essential oils can provide an answer.

One drop of **Roman chamomile** or one drop of **dill** or one drop of **mandarin** can be added to 15 ml of carrier oil and massaged gently into the baby's abdomen.

If the baby continues to cry, try a compress of Roman chamomile. Add one drop of Roman chamomile to a small amount of water in a bowl. Stir well and soak a flannel in the solution. Place the flannel on the baby's abdomen.

If the colic persists, the mother should consider her diet carefully. Perhaps the baby is allergic to the dairy foods that she is eating? It is also well worth the effort to take the baby to see a fully qualified osteopath who has experience in the cranial field with babies (see 'Taking it Further'.

Coughs and colds

Aromatherapy is an excellent way of preventing babies from picking up coughs and colds. If someone in the household has a cold, the baby can be protected by using essential oils in a diffuser or by using the plant spray method (see page 23). **Tea tree, eucalyptus** and **cajeput** are all excellent oils to diffuse.

You may also place a small bowl of boiling water under the baby's cot to which you have added one drop of cajeput/myrtle and one drop of tea tree.

One drop of **lavender** on a piece of cotton wool placed at the bottom of the crib or the cot will also help the baby to breathe and sleep more easily.

Cradle cap

'Cradle cap' is the term given to 'crusting' on the scalp. It is easy to relieve with essential oils. My favourite oil for this is **geranium**. Add one drop of geranium to 15 ml of sweet almond oil and massage *gently* on to the scalp. This mixture should be used daily until the cradle cap subsides.

Insomnia/restlessness

It is often difficult to get a baby into a sleeping routine which suits the parents. Some babies like to sleep in the day and wake up in the night. To establish a good pattern put one drop of **lavender** and one drop of **Roman chamomile** into a diffuser or vapouriser and light it or switch it on about half an hour before bedtime, ensuring that you close the bedroom door.

Alternatively, place a small bowl of boiling water under the cot to which you have added two drops of Roman chamomile.

Nappy rash

Nappy rash can be prevented and treated by essential oils. When you change the baby, avoid using chemically perfumed 'baby wipes'. Instead add one drop of **Roman chamomile** or **lavender** or **yarrow** to one pint of water and agitate the water thoroughly. With my two children I used to put a drop in the sink and dip them in to clean their bottoms. You can also add essential oils to a jar of pure organic skin cream or zinc and castor oil cream. Add approximately one drop per 15 g. To a 60 g jar of cream add two drops of Roman chamomile, one drop of lavender and one drop of yarrow. To a 100 g jar add two drops of Roman chamomile, two drops of lavender and two drops of yarrow.

Teething

Teething usually begins around four to six months although there are wide variations and it has been known for a baby to be born with teeth. Teething can be a painful experience for the baby and for the parents who often have to endure many sleepless nights. **Roman chamomile, lavender** and **yarrow** are three of the best essential oils for teething. Put one drop of any of the essential oils into an egg cup full of carrier oil. Stir the mixture well and using your finger or a cotton bud massage baby's gums and also massage externally on the affected side of the face.

Bach Flower Remedies for babies

The Bach Flower Remedies can be of enormous help to babies who usually respond much more rapidly to them than adults. They have not yet accumulated all the 'emotional baggage' which some adults carry around with them and the Remedies can get to work straightaway.

Star of Bethlehem should always be administered after a traumatic birth. Birth is a difficult enough journey without any complications. **Olive** is an essential remedy for the parents since it is indicated for weariness and exhaustion. I have never met parents who are not tired. The whole family should take **Walnut** to help them to adjust to the idea of a new baby in the house. **Chicory** is for sleepy, drowsy babies who are clingy and do not want to be left on their own. **Clematis** is for sleepy, drowsy babies who do not even bother to wake up for feeds. These babies have a 'far away' look in their eyes and appear to have no interest in this world. **Mimulus** can be prescribed for fearful, nervous babies who are easily startled and usually cry on awakening. **Vervain** can help overactive babies who seem unable to relax and have great difficulty in going to sleep.

Aromatherapy for children

Children also respond very rapidly to the effects of essential oils. Their innate powers of self-healing enable them to throw off toxins very quickly because their bodies are not impaired by years of bad diet, lack of exercise, negative thoughts, pollution and stress.

Essential oils should *never* be given internally to young children. You should not try to treat serious illnesses or indeed any illnesses which have not been diagnosed by a qualified medical practitioner. Suitable dilutions for children are:

Small children (1–5 years) 1–2 drops per 10 ml carrier oil in a massage; 2 drops in the bath (add to a teaspoon of carrier oil).
Juniors (5–12 years) 2–3 drops per 10 ml carrier oil in a massage; 3 – 4 drops in the bath (add to a teaspoon of carrier oil).
Adolescents (12 years +) 3 drops per 10 ml carrier oil in a massage; 4–5 drops in the bath.

Allergies (e.g. eczema)

Food allergies are very common in children and are responsible for many hyperactivity and behavioural problems. Children may be sensitive to additives and preservatives, as well as dairy foods, sugar and wheat.

Roman chamomile, lavender or **yarrow** can be added to the bath-water in the appropriate dilution. These oils may also be added to a pure organic skin cream or moisturising lotion and applied several times daily, depending upon the severity of the condition to ease discomfort, inflammation and itching. Essential oils such as **geranium, melissa, neroli, rose** and **sandalwood** will help if the allergy is stress-related, and should be added to the daily bath.

If possible the food(s) or other offending substances causing the reaction(s) should be isolated and eliminated.

Asthma

Asthma attacks are very frightening for young children and their parents. They can be related to allergies to food and environmental factors such as house-dust. Stress will increase the severity and frequency of the attacks.

Aromatherapy treatment is aimed at reducing the anxiety and improving the function of the lungs. Essential oils useful for asthma include **cypress, frankincense, lavender, marjoram, melissa, neroli, Roman chamomile** and **rose**. A blend of any of these oils can be massaged into the upper back and chest. Alternatively, put one drop of essential oil on a handkerchief or tissue and inhale deeply.

Asthma formulae

child (1–5 years)

1 drop lavender
1 drop Roman
  chamomile
} or
1 drop Roman
  chamomile
1 drop neroli
} diluted in
10 ml of
carrier oil

child (5–12 years)

1 drop frankincense
1 drop lavender
1 drop marjoram
} or
1 drop cypress
1 drop frankincense
1 drop Roman
  chamomile
} diluted in
10 ml of
carrier oil

Athlete's foot (tinea pedis)

This fungal infection found in between the toes is often picked up by children at swimming pools and in changing rooms. The skin becomes damp, flaky, itchy, spongy and white.

Useful essential oils include **cypress, lavender, lemon, tagetes** and **tea tree.** The child should be encouraged to have at least two footbaths daily, to which you have added one, or a combination, of the oils suggested above. One drop of lavender, one drop of tagetes and one drop of tea tree is an excellent combination. These essential oils may also be added to two teaspoons of carrier oil dabbed in between the toes.

The skin should be kept as dry as possible between the toes and only cotton or wool socks should be worn (not nylon or synthetic fibres).

Bruises

Immediately after a bump essential oils may be applied on an ice-cold compress. Add one drop of **lavender** and one drop of **Roman chamomile** to a small bowl of cold water. Use a flannel to soak up the solution, wring it out and apply to the affected area.

Burns

Hold the affected area under running cold water then apply a cold compress to which you have added two drops of pure essential oil of **lavender.** Other useful oils for burns include **Roman chamomile** and **yarrow.**

Colds and coughs

The anti-bacterial and anti-viral properties of essential oils are extremely effective when treating coughs and colds.

If the child has a **fever** then **lavender, Roman chamomile** and **tea tree** are beneficial. Place one drop of each into a small bowl of lukewarm water and sponge down the body and head until the fever subsides. Alternatively, make a cold compress to which you have added these oils, and place it on the back of the neck or forehead or wrap it around the feet.

For **coughs** massage the chest, throat and upper back using a blend containing the appropriate number of drops of essential oils chosen from **cajeput, cypress, eucalyptus, frankincense, lavender, myrtle, Roman chamomile, rosemary** or **tea tree**. These oils will help to fight the infection, expel the mucus, relieve bronchial spasm and induce relaxation.

Coughs and colds formulae

child (1–5 years)

1 drop lavender 1 drop tea tree	} 1 drop lavender 1 drop myrtle	} diluted in 10 ml of carrier oil

child (5–12 years)

1 drop cajeput 1 drop lavender 1 drop tea tree	} 1 drop frankincense 1 drop myrtle 1 drop Roman chamomile	} diluted in 10 ml of carrier oil

Cuts and grazes

It is very important to clean the area thoroughly to prevent any infection. Useful essential oils include **lavender, lemon** and **tea tree**. Bathe the wound with warm water to which you have added one drop of lavender plus one drop of tea tree. This will calm the child and will not sting as much as a proprietary antiseptic. If a dressing is needed, one drop of neat lavender on a sticking plaster will accelerate the healing process.

Digestive problems

Constipation in children can be caused by poor eating habits or even by stress. Encourage your children to eat plenty of fresh fruit and vegetables in preference to 'junk food' and to drink plenty of water and fruit juices to reduce dehydration of the stools. Straining should be avoided; do not put your children under pressure to 'perform' on the toilet.

Useful essential oils to treat constipation include **geranium, mandarin, marjoram, Roman chamomile, rosemary** and **spearmint**. The best method of application is to massage the abdomen daily, working in a clockwise direction.

Constipation formulae

child (1–5 years)

1 drop mandarin
1 drop Roman chamomile }

child (5–12 years)

1 drop mandarin
1 drop marjoram
1 drop spearmint } diluted in 10 ml of carrier oil

Diarrhoea may be caused by an infection, an allergy to food, certain drugs or by stress. It is vital to replace lost fluid to prevent dehydration. Avoid food but drink as much liquid as possible. If the diarrhoea persists then consult a medically qualified practitioner.

Useful essential oils for diarrhoea include **geranium, ginger, lavender, neroli, Roman chamomile** and **sandalwood**. A massage blend may be gently rubbed into the abdomen and compresses may be applied to help to alleviate pain.

Diarrhoea formulae

child (1–5 years)

1 drop lavender
1 drop neroli }

child (5–12 years)

1 drop ginger
1 drop neroli
1 drop Roman
  chamomile } diluted in 10 ml of carrier oil

Earache

Blend one drop of either **lavender** or **Roman chamomile** with a teaspoon of olive oil. Soak a piece of cotton wool in this mixture and place it in the ear. If pain is severe, rub any swollen glands, using the appropriate number of drops of lavender and Roman chamomile. If the earache is recurrent, visit an osteopath who specialises in children (see 'Taking it Further').

Head lice

Please refer to page 153.

Infectious diseases

Chicken-pox   Add **lavender** and **Roman chamomile** to the bath. Add either Roman chamomile and lavender or Roman chamomile and **tea tree** to moisturising lotion and massage.

Measles   Use **Roman chamomile** and **lavender** in oil or moisturising lotion and massage gently.

Mumps   Blend the appropriate number of drops into a massage oil using either **lavender, lemon** or **tea tree**.

Rubella (German measles)   Blend the appropriate number of drops into a massage oil using **lavender, Roman chamomile** or **tea tree**.

Whooping cough   Blend the appropriate number of drops for the child's age into a massage oil and rub the chest and add one drop to the child's pillow using either **cypress, lavender, rosemary** or **tea tree**.

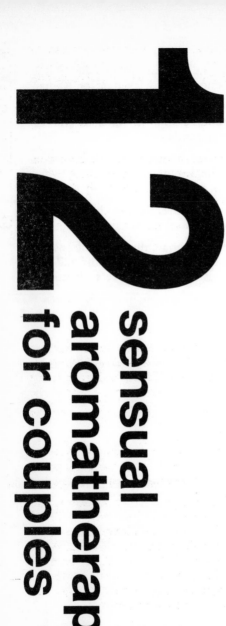

12
sensual
aromatherapy
for couples

In this chapter you will learn:

- how to make yourself more sexually attractive with essential oils
- how to enhance your love life
- how aromatherapy may help t[overcome sexual difficulties.

All of us have our own natural body scent and we can be attracted to another person by the way that he or she smells. Aromas can have erotic connotations. Sexual arousal causes the body to release all sorts of exotic odours – especially from the skin, breath and sexual organs. It is possible to enhance these odours by using essential oils to make ourselves more sexually attractive.

The aroma of a 'love potion' must of course suit both your tastes. Aroma preference is important when deciding which essential oils to blend together, as we are instinctively drawn to those essential oils which we need.

There are many ways of using essential oils to enhance your love life and to achieve sexual fulfilment.

Scenting

Scenting your lingerie

It is easy to perfume your own lingerie. When you are washing your delicate and seductive items by hand, just add two drops of essential oil to the final rinse. If you are washing by machine then put four drops to a small amount of water and add to the final rinse in the softener section.

Sensual oils for your lingerie

Bergamot, geranium, neroli and **ylang ylang** are all excellent choices. It is advisable not to use absolutes or the thick heavy oils to perfume your lingerie as they may stain the fabric.

You can also perfume your lingerie in your chest of drawers and in your wardrobe. Sprinkle about six drops of essential oils of **rose, myrtle, jasmine, neroli, bergamot, geranium, ylang ylang, patchouli, frankincense** or **sandalwood** or whatever your preference is on to cotton-wool balls and place them in greaseproof bags. Prick holes in the bags to allow the wonderful fragrances to permeate into your clothing. Place these bags into your drawers or hang them up inside your wardrobe.

Beautiful aromatic silk bags make wonderful presents. Cut out a circle of silk and stitch around the circumference with a thick thread. Place a cotton-wool ball which has been sprinkled with essential oils into the centre of the silk circle. Gather up the thread so that the cotton-wool ball(s) is enclosed by the silk.

Sew on a piece of thin ribbon so that you can hang up your pomander. Particularly suitable essential oils would be: **frankincense, patchouli, rose, jasmine, vetivert** and **ylang ylang** as these aromas will last a long time.

You can even make your own drawer liners to perfume your clothes. Sprinkle six drops of essential oil on to squares of blotting paper or any absorbent pieces of paper.

Scenting your bedlinen

Scented bedlinen is sensual and it is easy to do. There are several methods:

1 Put four drops of essential oil into a small amount of water and add to the softener section of your washing machine for the final rinse.
2 Fill a small plant spray with spring water, add ten drops of the essential oils of your own choice and then spray the bottom sheet lightly.
3 Put a few drops of your chosen essential oils on to cotton-wool balls or on to pieces of absorbent, natural material and place them between the sheets in your airing cupboard, or inside your pillow case.

Scenting your bedroom

A clay burner or radiator fragrancer is the perfect way to create a romantic and sensual environment. Put a few teaspoons of water into the loose bowl on top of your clay burner and sprinkle six drops into it. Light the night light to allow the oils to diffuse into the air.

Suggested recipes for your burner:

2 drops rose		2 drops jasmine		2 drops benzoin		2 drops clary sage
2 drops geranium	or	2 drops patchouli	or	2 drops rose	or	2 drops frankincense
2 drops sandalwood		2 drops ylang ylang		2 drops neroli		2 drops ylang ylang

For more masculine aroma try:

$$\left.\begin{array}{l} 3 \text{ drops} \\ \quad \text{cedarwood} \\ 3 \text{ drops} \\ \quad \text{sandalwood} \end{array}\right\}or \left.\begin{array}{l} 2 \text{ drops} \\ \quad \text{black pepper} \\ 2 \text{ drops} \\ \quad \text{ylang ylang} \\ 2 \text{ drops} \\ \quad \text{lemon/} \\ \quad \text{mandarin} \end{array}\right\}or \left.\begin{array}{l} 3 \text{ drops} \\ \quad \text{benzoin} \\ 3 \text{ drops} \\ \quad \text{sandalwood} \end{array}\right\}or \left.\begin{array}{l} 2 \text{ drops} \\ \quad \text{bergamot} \\ 2 \text{ drops} \\ \quad \text{ginger} \\ 2 \text{ drops} \\ \quad \text{vetivert} \end{array}\right\}$$

Candles are also perfect for scenting your bedroom and creating a romantic scene. Light your candle and wait until the wax has slightly melted and then *carefully* put one to two drops of essential oil into the melted wax, taking care to avoid the wick. The following suggestions may be useful:

- To a pink candle add essential oil of rose to encourage new love, romance and gentleness;
- To a red candle add ylang ylang to induce passion and sexuality;
- To a violet candle add frankincense to add an air of mystery.

Massage

Massage is an excellent way of arousing your partner and it is not necessary to have had a training in massage to achieve the desired effect. Just follow your instincts. Pay particular attention to the abdominal area, especially the area from the navel to the pubis and the low back and buttocks. There are some effective points for boosting sexual energy and heightening sexual response.

To set the scene, scent your room with one of the recipes already suggested and light a few candles around the room. Refer to Chapter 05 in this book and my other book in this series *Teach Yourself Massage* for specific massage techniques.

The following essential oils are ideal for increasing sexual desire: **benzoin, bergamot, black pepper, cinnamon, clary sage, frankincense, ginger, jasmine, melissa, myrtle, neroli, palmarosa, patchouli, petitgrain, rose, sandalwood, vetivert** and **ylang ylang.**

Suggested massage blends

For women:		For men:	
2 drops jasmine 2 drops rose 3 drops sandalwood 2 drops ylang ylang	} or	2 drops clary sage 2 drops ginger or black pepper 3 drops sandalwood 2 drops ylang ylang	} diluted in 10 ml of carrier oil

Sexual difficulties

Vaginal dryness

Lack of vaginal secretion can make intercourse difficult, uncomfortable or even impossible. Some of the factors affecting secretion include hormone imbalance such as experienced at the menopause, the contraceptive pill or negative emotions.

A simple solution to this problem is to apply a small amount of jojoba to the vagina. However, this is only a temporary remedy. For the long term, essential oils which increase vaginal secretions (especially those that imitate the hormone oestrogen) should be used in the bath (6 drops) or in massage blends (3–4 drops to 10 ml of carrier oil).

Take a daily bath with one of the formulae and use the massage recipe every day for a week and you should notice an increase in secretion.

Bath formulae to overcome vaginal dryness

| 2 drops clary sage
1 drop geranium
3 drops rose | } or | 2 drops fennel
2 drops geranium
2 drops lavender | } or | 1 drop melissa
2 drops neroli
3 drops
  sandalwood | } |

Alternatively, use any of the oils mentioned in the formula singularly.

Massage formula

| 2 drops clary sage
2 drops fennel
2 drops rose
2 drops sandalwood | } | diluted in
30 ml
of
carrier oil |

Impotence

A temporary state of impotence can happen to any man. The cause may be physical or emotional exhaustion, nervous tension, lack of confidence or a symptom of illness. Some drugs can affect the libido such as valium and librium. Whatever the reason the following essential oils are invaluable. Choose any three or use one of my suggested recipes: **amyris, basil, black pepper, cardamon, celery, clary sage, coriander, cinnamon leaf, cumin, geranium, ginger, jasmine, lavender, patchouli, rose, rosemary, rosewood, sage, sandalwood, thyme, violet leaf, ylang ylang.**

Massage formulae for impotence

| 1 drop cinnamon
1 drop coriander
2 drops ginger
1 drop
  rosemary | or | 1 drop clary sage
2 drops ginger
1 drop jasmine
2 drops
  sandalwood | or | 2 drops black
  pepper
2 drops ginger
2 drops
  rosewood | diluted
in 15 ml
of carrier
oil |

Massage one of these formulae into your partner paying particular attention to the lower back, the upper abdominal area and upper thighs. Make sure that you avoid the genitals. Apply the oils for approximately ten days and have a daily bath using about four drops of ginger and two drops of black pepper.

For men who suffer with **premature ejaculation** the following blend should be effective:

| 1 drop benzoin
2 drops marjoram
1 drop vetivert | diluted in
30 ml of
carrier oil |

Bach Flower Remedies

The word 'impotence' has an enormous stigma attached to it and can put a strain on a marriage or partnership, resulting in endless rows and eventually can cause a rift in a relationship. Since impotence is often of emotional origin the Bach Flower Remedies are invaluable.

Larch is a wonderful Remedy for boosting a lack of confidence and feelings of inadequacy; **White Chestnut** is useful for the worries which a man has concerning his virility; **Olive** is essential for exhaustion whether physical or emotional; **Mimulus** is excellent for fear of failure.

Frigidity

There are many factors which contribute to a lack of sexual response. The hormone which is responsible for the sex drive in both men and women is testosterone. Levels of testosterone vary not only between males and females but also among women. Those with high testosterone levels have a strong sexual appetite. Anxiety, or fear, perhaps from some traumatic experience in the past, can actually cause levels of this hormone to deplete. Fatigue and stress due to pressures with work, money or family will also lower the sex drive.

Boredom and lack of sexual satisfaction can also result in frigidity. Some women have never experienced an orgasm. If a man takes his partner for granted and does not indulge in any foreplay then this will eventually lead to sexual unresponsiveness or even aversion.

Lack of libido may also be caused by stress and exhaustion. If a woman is working and has several children to look after no wonder she loses her sex drive.

Essential oils to combat frigidity

Clary sage, ginger, jasmine, neroli, rose, sandalwood, and ylang ylang are all effective. Any of these oils can be used in your daily bath to stimulate and renew your interest in sex.

Massage formulae for frigidity

2 drops clary sage		1 drop ginger		diluted in
2 drops jasmine	or	2 drops rose		30 ml of
2 drops ylang ylang		2 drops ylang ylang		carrier oil

Use one of the recipes above for about ten days. The oils should be applied particularly to the upper thighs, abdomen and lower back.

Bach Flower Remedies

For the majority of women frigidity is of an emotional origin and the Bach Flower Remedies can be helpful. If the problem arises from exhaustion then **Olive** is the recommended Remedy. For fear of sex **Mimulus** can help to ease the problem. **Honeysuckle** is beneficial where the woman has suffered a traumatic experience in the past such as rape. If this has led to a sense of being 'dirty' and 'contaminated', then **Crab Apple** would be beneficial. **Wild Rose** is helpful for those who suffer from boredom and have a submissive approach. **Willow** is invaluable for the anger and resentment which the woman may experience if her partner is unable to satisfy her needs.

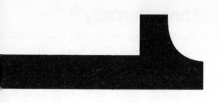

13

spiritual/
vibrational
aromatherapy

In this chapter you will learn:
- how to use aromatherapy on a spiritual level
- essential oils for balancing the charkas.

What is spiritual aromatherapy?

It is the use of essential oils in order to affect the spirit. In vibrational aromatherapy it is not even necessary to touch the physical body. Instead one works off the body in the aura using a *minute* amount of essential oil – just one drop will suffice.

What is the aura?

The idea of an aura may seem strange or even ridiculous to you. However, we are not just a physical body. We are completely surrounded by the subtle energy bodies which make up our human energy field (aura). The size and shape of the aura varies enormously from one person to another. It is filled with many different colours which constantly change depending upon our emotions and well-being. Some are able to see the aura and the colour changes. In our everyday language we talk of being 'green with envy' or 'red with rage' and these lucky individuals would actually be able to 'see' this occurring!

I believe that we can all at least sense the aura. Try the following exercise. Hold your hands out in front of you, palms facing and gently touching each other. Close your eyes and very slowly move your hands a few inches away from each other. Gradually bring them back towards each other. Repeat this several times. You will feel as if there is 'something' in the space between your hands. This is your energy field! Now try to sense another person's aura. Ask a friend to sit on a chair. Close your eyes and hold your hands a few inches above their head. Slowly move your hands down following the outline of the body and notice any tingling, feelings of warmth, coldness or any other sensations. Ask your friend if they have experienced anything. Amazing isn't it?

What are chakras?

The word 'chakra' is a Sanskrit word which means 'wheel', 'disc' or 'circle'. The chakras are like constantly revolving wheels of energy which penetrate both the aura and the physical body. They can also be visualised as lotus flowers – each chakra having a different number of petals. The chakras act as a bridge between the physical body and the subtle bodies. There are seven major chakras which I shall describe briefly.

Crown Chakra

Third Eye/Brow Chakra

Throat Chakra

Heart Chakra

Solar Plexus Chakra

Abdomen/Sacral Chakra

Base/Root Chakra

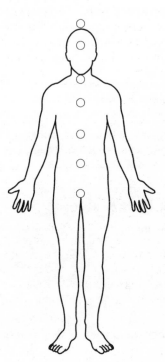

Chakra One: Base/Root Chakra

Sanskrit name:	Muladhara
Meaning:	Root/support
Location:	Base of the spine in the perineum between the anus and genitals
Colour:	Red
Element:	Earth
Function:	Survival, grounding, security. It connects us with the physical world – the earth
Glands connected with:	Adrenals or some say gonads (i.e. testes/ovaries)
Petals:	4
Sound:	LAM

Physical imbalances include: the feet, ankles, knees, thighs, low back problems, sciatica, constipation and haemorrhoids. Lethargy (physical and mental) could result or an inability to sit still.

Psychological imbalances include: feelings of 'spaciness', inability to ground oneself, insecurity.

Chakra Two: Abdomen/Sacral Chakra

Sanskrit name:	Svadhisthana
Meaning:	Seat of vital force/sweetness
Location:	Lower abdomen
Colour:	Orange
Element:	Water
Function:	Desire, sexuality
Glands connected with:	Ovaries/testes (Or some say spleen)
Petals:	6
Sound:	VAM

Physical imbalances include: Malfunction of male/female sexual organs, impotence, frigidity, kidney or bladder problems, prostate problems and digestive problems.

Psychological imbalances include: Sexual perversion, promiscuity, possessiveness, greed.

Chakra Three: Solar Plexus Chakra/Navel Chakra

Sanskrit name:	Manipura
Meaning:	Power chakra, lustrous gem
Location:	Between the navel and the solar plexus
Colour:	Yellow
Element:	Fire
Function:	Power
Glands connected with:	Pancreas or some say adrenals
Petals:	10
Sound:	RAM

Physical imbalances include: Digestive problems such as stomach ulcers, diabetes, hypoglycaemia, allergies, anorexia, bulimia, chronic fatigue.

Psychological imbalances include: Low self-esteem, nervous exhaustion, addictions, mood swings, inability to relax.

Chakra Four: Heart Chakra

Sanskrit name:	Anahata
Meaning:	Unstruck
Location:	Centre of chest
Colour:	Green (also pink)
Element:	Air
Function:	Unconditional love
Glands connected with:	Thymus
Petals:	12
Sound:	YAM

Physical imbalances include: Asthma, blood pressure and circulatory problems, heart problems, respiratory disorders, poor immune system.

Psychological imbalances include: Depression, inability to love oneself and others, self destructive, lack of compassion, inability to forgive.

Chakra Five: Throat Chakra

Sanskrit name:	Visshuda
Meaning:	Purification
Location:	Throat
Colour:	Blue
Element:	Sound/ether
Function:	Communication/creativity
Glands connected with:	Thyroid
Petals:	16
Sound:	HAM

Physical imbalances: Throat problems, thyroid/parathyroid problems, neck and shoulder problems, stuttering, and non-stop verbal chatter.

Psychological imbalances: Inability to express oneself, blocked creativity.

Chakra Six: Third Eye Chakra

Sanskrit name:	Ajna
Meaning:	To command, to know
Location:	Centre of forehead
Colour:	Indigo
Element:	Light
Function:	Intuition
Glands connected with:	Pituitary or some say pineal
Petals:	2 (the two physical eyes surrounding the third eye). Some say 96 (2 × 48)
Sound:	OM

Physical imbalance: Eye/visual disorders, headaches, dizziness, nightmares.

Psychological imbalance: Extreme confusion, hallucinations, living in a fantasy world, lack of intuition.

Chakra Seven: Crown Chakra

Sanskrit name:	Sahasrara
Meaning:	Thousandfold
Location:	Crown of head (Anterior fontanelle of a newborn baby)
Colour:	Violet
Element:	Thought, knowing
Function:	Understanding/bliss/enlightenment
Glands connected with:	Pineal or some say pituitary
Petals:	1000
Sound:	Silent OM or silence

Physical imbalance: Epilepsy, Alzheimer's, Parkinson's disease, memory disorders.

Psychological imbalance: Fear of opening up to spiritual levels, closed mind.

Balancing the Chakras

Essential oils have the ability to unblock and balance the chakras and to help you along your spiritual path to enlightenment. I have listed some suggestions:

Base/Root Chakra

Oils to earth and ground such as benzoin, patchouli, vetivert.

Abdomen/Sacral Chakra

Aphrodisiac oils such as jasmine, neroli, rose, sandalwood, ylang ylang. Anaphrodisiac oils such as marjoram.

Solar Plexus/Navel Chakra

Oils to relax, balance mood swings, protect the solar plexus and increase confidence such as benzoin, chamomile, clary sage, geranium, jasmine, juniper (cleanses), lavender, lemon, mandarin, melissa, neroli, palmarosa, sage (protects), yarrow (protects).

Heart Chakra

Oils to open up and heal the heart such as benzoin, bergamot, geranium, jasmine, lime, mandarin, melissa, neroli, rose, ylang ylang.

Throat Chakra

Oils to encourage communication and creativity such as blue chamomile, black pepper, eucalyptus, ginger, jasmine, and myrrh.

Brow Chakra

Oils to encourage intuition and to clarify the mind such as basil, black pepper, carrot seed, clary sage, fennel, ginger, peppermint and rosemary.

Crown Chakra

Oils to open up the mind to spiritual levels such as cedarwood, frankincense, linden blossom, neroli, and rosewood.

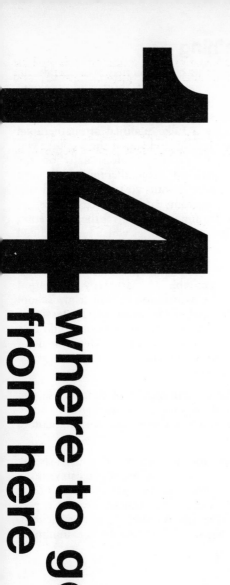

14

where to go from here

In this chapter you will learn:
- how to select a suitable aromatherapy college
- what to expect from a professional aromatherapy consultation.

Professional training

If you have been inspired by this book you may want to take an aromatherapy course. There are many short and weekend courses available which will give you the skills to help your friends and relations with simple problems. Please check any course you go on is run by a fully qualified aromatherapist (unfortunately many are not). Any weekend or short course will *not*, however, enable you to practise professionally on the general public. A fully qualified aromatherapist will have studied for anything from nine months to two years and will have a sound knowledge of anatomy and physiology, as well as massage and essential oils. Training also involves the completion of at least ten comprehensive case-histories which have included over sixty treatments.

You should check that the aromatherapy establishment you choose is accredited to a reputable aromatherapy association (see 'Taking it Further'). The association to which my school belongs is The International Federation of Professional Aromatherapists (IFPA). The principal of the school should be a qualified teacher, preferably recognised by the Department of Education and Science, and should have at least five years' clinical aromatherapy experience.

You should also check that on completion of your course you will be adequately insured to practise aromatherapy. Some schools issue a certificate which is a worthless, and sometimes very expensive, piece of paper.

The best way to choose an aromatherapy college is by recommendation. If you are at all unsure, ask if you can visit the school or college to look round, and perhaps see some of the former students' coursework and case histories. Do not expect to receive identical aromatherapy training from every school. Some schools will offer topics in addition to the minimum requirements.

An aromatherapy consultation

If after reading this book, you wish to try some aromatherapy treatments for yourself it is important to find a trained therapist so that you are not disappointed. The best way of finding a good aromatherapist is, again, by recommendation. You may well have to wait a while for the initial consultation (my own practice is booked up months in advance, and I have a long waiting list).

Do not be afraid to ask questions when you telephone to book your consultation. Ask if the therapist belongs to a professional association and check that he/she is properly insured.

The initial consultation can take up to one-and-a-half hours, although a very experienced practitioner will probably need less time. The first thirty minutes will be taken up by a series of detailed questions which are necessary if the therapist is to make an accurate evaluation of the patient. A skilled therapist will try to find out the cause of your problems rather than merely treating your symptoms. After the aromatherapist has made the initial assessment the essential oils will be selected. The blend which is chosen must match the individual's needs in order to benefit him/her holistically. All aspects of you as a person are considered – physical, emotional and spiritual.

The aromatherapy massage consists of a variety of techniques, once again tailored to your individual needs. A 'standard' form of aromatherapy massage, in my view, is unacceptable – how can the same aromatherapy treatment be suitable for everyone?

At the end of the treatment, you should experience a sense of deep relaxation. It is possible, although not inevitable, that you will have some reactions as a result of the aromatherapy treatment, due to the release of toxins. Any reaction should be viewed as positive and desirable, since this is indicative of your body's innate capacity for self-healing and shows that the essential oils are working.

The frequency of your bowel movements may increase, and your stools may also build up in bulk and volume. This is excellent as it is an indication that your body is casting aside its rubbish. It may be necessary to urinate more frequently after a treatment, especially if you have been suffering from fluid retention. You might develop a cold, particularly if your nasal passages and the bronchial tubes need unblocking. You may even experience emotional changes or develop more positive changes in your attitude to life. But do not worry – you will not experience all of these reactions at once and, any that you do, will be only temporary. However, you may not experience any reactions at all. Most patients feel marvellous after a treatment and report an improved sense of well-being and an increase in vitality. Their only complaint is that after one treatment they are thoroughly addicted to aromatherapy.

You may be given advice to carry out at home. The aromatherapist may give you a massage blend or some essential oils to add to your daily bath. You may also be given dietary advice.

All in all, an aromatherapy treatment should be a highly pleasurable experience. I have tried a wide range of complementary therapies and I am totally committed to my monthly aromatherapy treatments, which I find beneficial. Enjoy your aromatherapy and let it become part of your everyday life!

Circulatory/Immune Systems

Aids Chamomile, lavender, lemon, tea tree, thyme

anaemia Black pepper, carrot seed, chamomile, lemon, lime, peppermint, rosemary, thyme

arteriosclerosis Black pepper, cedarwood, ginger, juniper, lemon, rosemary, yarrow

chilblains Black pepper, ginger, lemon

fever Black pepper, chamomile, eucalyptus, ginger, juniper, lavender, peppermint

glandular fever Cypress, lavender, lemon, tea tree, thyme

haemorrhoids Cypress, geranium, juniper, myrrh, yarrow

heart *False angina*: Neroli. *Irregular heartbeat (tachycardia)*: Marjoram, melissa, petitgrain, sandalwood, ylang ylang. *Tonic*: Lavender, marjoram, neroli, rose

high blood pressure Clary sage, lavender, lemon, marjoram, melissa, neroli, yarrow, ylang ylang

high cholesterol Cedarwood, ginger, juniper, lemon, rosemary, thyme

immune system booster Carrot seed, chamomile, lavender, lemon, lemongrass, mandarin, petitgrain, tea tree, thyme, vetivert

low blood pressure Rosemary, sage, thyme

lymphatic congestion Carrot seed, cedarwood, cypress, fennel, grapefruit, juniper, mandarin, rosemary

M.E. (Myalgic encephalomyelitis) Cypress, grapefruit, lavender, lemongrass, rosemary, rosewood, tea tree, thyme

palpitations Clary sage, lavender, neroli, petitgrain, rose, rosemary, ylang ylang

poor circulation Benzoin, black pepper, carrot seed, cedarwood, cypress, eucalyptus, ginger, lemon, lemongrass, lime, mandarin, marjoram, rosemary, thyme

varicose veins Cypress, geranium, ginger, lemon, neroli, tea tree, yarrow

Digestive System

anorexia Bergamot, carrot seed, fennel, lavender, neroli, palmarosa, thyme

appetite balancer Fennel, patchouli

bulimia Bergamot, geranium, jasmine, lavender, neroli, rose

candida Tea tree

colic Bergamot, black pepper, chamomile, clary sage, fennel, juniper, lavender, lemongrass, marjoram, peppermint

colitis Bergamot, black pepper, chamomile, lavender, lemongrass, neroli, rosemary

constipation Black pepper, carrot seed, fennel, ginger, marjoram, patchouli, rose, rosemary, thyme

diabetes Eucalyptus, geranium, juniper

diarrhoea Black pepper, cajeput, chamomile, cypress, eucalyptus, geranium, ginger, lavender, lemon, mandarin, myrrh, neroli (stress induced), patchouli, petitgrain, peppermint, rosemary, sandalwood

fistula (anal) Lavender

flatulence Basil, bergamot, black pepper, carrot seed, chamomile, fennel, ginger, juniper, lavender, lemon, lemongrass, mandarin, marjoram, myrrh, neroli, peppermint, rosemary, thyme

food poisoning Black pepper, fennel, grapefruit, juniper, rosemary

gall bladder Bergamot, chamomile, geranium, grapefruit, lemon, mandarin, peppermint, rose, rosemary

hangover Fennel, juniper, rosemary

heartburn Black pepper, lemon (gastric antacid), lime

hiccoughs Basil, fennel, mandarin

indigestion Basil, bergamot, chamomile, cajeput, fennel, ginger, juniper, lavender, lemongrass, lime, mandarin, marjoram, melissa, myrrh, neroli (nervous), peppermint, rosemary

I.B.S. (Irritable bowel syndrome) Carrot seed, chamomile, ginger, myrrh, patchouli, petitgrain

liver Carrot seed, chamomile, cypress, geranium, grapefruit, lavender, lemon, mandarin, melissa, peppermint, rose, rosemary

loss of appetite Bergamot, black pepper, chamomile, fennel, ginger, juniper, lime, palmarosa, peppermint, thyme

nausea and vomiting Basil, black pepper, chamomile, fennel, ginger, lavender, melissa, peppermint

obesity Fennel, grapefruit, juniper, lemon, rosemary

sluggish digestion Black pepper, fennel, ginger, grapefruit, juniper, lemon, peppermint

spleen Chamomile

stomach pains Chamomile, fennel, ginger, lavender, marjoram, melissa, peppermint, rosemary

stomach ulcers Chamomile, lemon, marjoram

travel sickness Ginger, peppermint

worms and intestinal parasites Bergamot, chamomile, eucalyptus, geranium, juniper, lavender, myrrh, rosemary, tea tree, thyme

Genito-Urinary System

childbirth Clary sage, jasmine, lavender, neroli, palmarosa

cystitis Bergamot, cajeput, eucalyptus, frankincense, geranium, juniper, lavender, palmarosa, sandalwood, tea tree, yarrow

difficulty in passing urine Juniper

discharges Bergamot, lavender, marjoram, myrrh, rose, rosemary, sandalwood, tea tree, thyme

enuresis (bed-wetting) Cypress

excessive sexual impulses Marjoram

fluid retention Benzoin, carrot seed, cedarwood, chamomile, cypress, eucalyptus, fennel, geranium, juniper, lavender, lemon, lemongrass, rosemary, sandalwood, thyme, yarrow

frigidity and impotence Clary sage, ginger, jasmine, neroli, rose, sandalwood, ylang ylang

insufficiency of milk in nursing mothers Fennel, jasmine, lemongrass

itching (vaginal) Bergamot, cedarwood, chamomile, tea tree

kidney infections and stones Chamomile, eucalyptus, fennel, geranium, juniper, lemon, sandalwood

menopause Carrot seed, chamomile, cypress, fennel, frankincense, geranium, jasmine, lavender, neroli, rose

menstruation: *Heavy blood loss*: Chamomile, cypress, geranium, rose, yarrow. *Irregular*: Chamomile, melissa, marjoram, rose, yarrow. *Painful*: Chamomile, cajeput, clary sage, cypress, jasmine, juniper, lavender, marjoram, myrrh, peppermint, rose, rosemary, yarrow. *Scanty*: Chamomile, clary sage, fennel, juniper, lavender, myrrh, peppermint, rose, rosemary, thyme, yarrow.

oestrogen (stimulates body to produce) Fennel

PMS Chamomile, cypress, geranium, lavender, marjoram, neroli, rose

prostate enlargement Jasmine, juniper

sterility Geranium, melissa, rose

thrush Bergamot, eucalyptus, frankincense, lavender, lemon, myrrh, tea tree

tonic for the womb Clary sage, jasmine, rose

urinary infections Bergamot, cajeput, eucalyptus, juniper, sandalwood, thyme

Head Disorders

catarrh Basil, cedarwood, eucalyptus, black pepper, frankincense, lavender, lemon, lime, myrrh, tea tree

cold sores Bergamot, chamomile, lavender, lemon, melissa, tea tree

earache Basil, chamomile, lavender

fainting and vertigo Basil, black pepper, lavender, peppermint, rosemary

gum infections (e.g. gingivitis) Chamomile, lemon, myrrh, tea tree, thyme

hair and scalp *Dandruff*: Carrot seed, chamomile, cypress, juniper, lavender, lemon, patchouli, tea tree, thyme. *Dry*: Carrot seed, geranium, lavender, palmarosa, rosemary, rosewood, sandalwood. *Lice*: Bergamot, eucalyptus, geranium, lavender, lemon, rosemary, tea tree. *Loss of hair*: Chamomile, cedarwood, clary sage, frankincense, geranium, ginger, lavender, rosemary, yarrow. *Oily*: Bergamot, cedarwood, clary sage, cypress, frankincense, geranium, lemon, lemongrass, juniper, rosemary, thyme, yarrow. *Sensitive scalp*: Chamomile, lavender

headaches and migraine Basil, chamomile, lavender, marjoram, peppermint, rosemary

loss of smell Rosemary

mouth infections and ulcers Lemon, myrrh, tea tree, thyme

nasal polyps Basil

neuralgia Basil, black pepper, chamomile, eucalyptus, geranium, peppermint

rhinitis and sinusitis Basil, cajeput, eucalyptus, lavender, peppermint, tea tree, thyme

toothache Cajeput, chamomile, peppermint

Muscular/Joint Disorders

aches and pains Black pepper, cajeput, chamomile, eucalyptus, frankincense, ginger, juniper, lavender, lemon, lemongrass, lime, marjoram, peppermint, rosemary, thyme

arthritis Basil, benzoin, black pepper, cajeput, chamomile, eucalyptus, ginger, grapefruit, juniper, lavender, lemon, marjoram, peppermint, rosemary, thyme, vetivert

bruises Chamomile, geranium, lavender, marjoram

cramp Basil, chamomile, ginger, lavender, marjoram, rosemary, vetivert

fibrositis Benzoin, black pepper, eucalyptus, lavender, peppermint, rosemary

gout Basil, Benzoin, cajeput, chamomile, grapefruit, juniper, lemon, lime, rosemary, thyme

inflammation Chamomile, lavender, yarrow

lack of muscle tone Black pepper, lavender, lemongrass, rosemary

rheumatism Basil, black pepper, cajeput, chamomile, eucalyptus, frankincense, ginger, juniper, lavender, lemon, lime, marjoram, peppermint, rosemary, thyme, vetivert

sprains and strains Black pepper, cajeput, chamomile, eucalyptus, ginger, lavender, lemongrass, marjoram, peppermint, rosemary, vetivert, yarrow

stiffness Black pepper, chamomile, eucalyptus, grapefruit, lavender, marjoram, palmarosa, rosemary

Nervous System

alcoholism Fennel, juniper (detoxify)

anger Chamomile, cypress, yarrow, ylang ylang

anorexia nervosa Basil, benzoin, bergamot, geranium, jasmine, juniper, lavender, mandarin, marjoram, neroli, patchouli, sandalwood, thyme, ylang ylang

apathy and lethargy Ginger, jasmine, lemongrass, lime, myrrh, patchouli, rosemary

change Cypress (enables you to accept it), frankincense (enables you to move on)

coldness Benzoin, black pepper, frankincense, marjoram, rose

comfort Benzoin, black pepper, cypress, marjoram, rose, rosewood

confidence (lack of) Ginger, jasmine

courage Black pepper, fennel, ginger

depression Basil, bergamot, chamomile, clary sage, geranium, grapefruit, jasmine, lavender, lemongrass, lime, mandarin, melissa, neroli, patchouli, rose, sandalwood, thyme, ylang-ylang

exhaustion Benzoin (mental, emotional, physical), clary sage (nervous, physical, sexual), eucalyptus, juniper (emotional and nervous depletion), lavender, thyme

fearful Clary sage, jasmine, lavender, melissa, neroli, frankincense, sandalwood, ylang ylang

frigidity and impotence Clary sage, ginger, jasmine, neroli, patchouli, peppermint, rose, rosewood, sandalwood, ylang-ylang

grief Benzoin, cypress, frankincense, mandarin, marjoram, melissa, neroli, rose

hysteria and panic Chamomile, clary sage, lavender, melissa, neroli, marjoram

inability to concentrate Basil, lemon, peppermint, rosemary

indecision Basil, carrot seed, patchouli

insomnia Chamomile, lavender, mandarin, marjoram, neroli, rose, sandalwood, ylang ylang

irritability Chamomile, cypress, lavender, thyme, yarrow

jealousy Rose

loneliness Benzoin, rose

memory (poor) Basil, black pepper, ginger, juniper, rosemary, thyme

mental fatigue (clears the mind) Basil, peppermint, rosemary

mood swings Chamomile, geranium, lavender

negativity Jasmine, juniper, mandarin, palmarosa

nervous tension Basil, cedarwood, clary sage, cypress, geranium, grapefruit, mandarin, marjoram, neroli, palmarosa, patchouli, petitgrain, rose, sandalwood

neuralgia Basil, black pepper, chamomile, eucalyptus, geranium, peppermint

obsessions Frankincense, vetivert

over sensitivity Basil, black pepper, chamomile, cypress, geranium, lavender

resentment Grapefruit

sadness Benzoin, jasmine, rose

sedative Bergamot, chamomile, clary sage, frankincense, marjoram, sandalwood, vetivert

self-obsession Rose

shock Benzoin, mandarin, neroli, peppermint, rose, ylang ylang

Respiratory System

asthma Basil, benzoin, cajeput, cypress, eucalyptus, frankincense, lavender, lemon, lime, melissa, myrrh, peppermint, rosemary, thyme

breath (fast) Frankincense, lavender

breath (shortness of) Fennel, frankincense, lavender

bronchitis Basil, benzoin, cajeput, cypress, eucalyptus, fennel, frankincense, ginger, lavender, lemon, lime, melissa, myrrh, peppermint rosemary, sandalwood, tea tree, thyme

catarrh Basil, benzoin, black pepper, cajeput, cedarwood, eucalyptus, frankincense, ginger, lavender, lemon, myrrh, rosemary, sandalwood, tea tree

coughs and colds Benzoin, bergamot, black pepper, cajeput, eucalyptus, frankincense, ginger, grapefruit, lavender, lemon, lime, melissa, myrrh, peppermint, rosemary, rosewood, sandalwood, tea tree, thyme

cough (whooping) Cypress, lavender, rosemary, thyme

emphysema Eucalyptus, frankincense

flu Benzoin, bergamot, black pepper, eucalyptus, fennel, frankincense, ginger, grapefruit, lavender, lemon, lime, peppermint, rosemary, rosewood, tea tree

hoarseness and loss of voice Myrrh, sandalwood

laryngitis Benzoin, bergamot, cajeput, eucalyptus, lemon, myrrh, sandalwood

sinusitis Basil, cajeput, eucalyptus, lavender, lemon, tea tree, thyme

tonsillitis and throat infections Benzoin, bergamot, cajeput, eucalyptus, geranium, ginger, lavender, lemon, lime, myrrh, rosewood, sandalwood

Skin

acne Bergamot, carrot seed, cedarwood, chamomile, grapefruit, juniper, lavender, lemongrass, lime, mandarin, patchouli, palmarosa, peppermint, rosemary, sandalwood, tea tree, yarrow

ageing skin Clary sage, frankincense, lavender, lemon, myrrh, neroli, patchouli, rose, rosemary

allergy Chamomile, lavender, melissa, patchouli

athlete's foot Lavender, lemongrass, myrrh, patchouli, tea tree

bleeding Geranium

boils and carbuncles Bergamot, chamomile, lavender, lemon, lime, rosemary, tea tree, thyme

broken capillaries Chamomile, cypress, frankincense, lemon, parsley seed, neroli, rose, sandalwood

bruises Chamomile, fennel, geranium, lavender, marjoram

burns Chamomile, eucalyptus, lavender, geranium, yarrow

cellulite Cedarwood, cypress, fennel, geranium, grapefruit, juniper, lemon, lime, rosemary, sage

chapped and cracked skin Benzoin, myrrh, palmarosa, patchouli, sandalwood, tea tree

combination skin Geranium, lavender, neroli

cuts Eucalyptus, geranium, lavender, lemon, tea tree

dermatitis Benzoin, juniper, lavender, myrrh, patchouli, peppermint, rosemary

dry skin Benzoin, carrot seed, chamomile, clary sage, frankincense, geranium, jasmine, lavender, neroli, palmarosa, rose, rosewood, sandalwood, vetivert, ylang ylang

eczema Bergamot, geranium, juniper, lavender, myrrh, palmarosa, patchouli, rosemary, yarrow

herpes Bergamot, eucalyptus, lavender, lemon, lime, melissa, tea tree

inflamed, red, irritated skin Benzoin, chamomile, clary sage, geranium, lavender, myrrh, neroli, patchouli, peppermint, rose

mature skin Carrot seed, clary sage, frankincense, geranium, jasmine, lavender, myrrh, neroli, palmarosa, patchouli, rose, rosewood, sandalwood, yarrow

measles (and other infectious diseases) Bergamot, eucalyptus, geranium, lemon, lemongrass, rosemary, tea tree

oily and open pores Bergamot, cajeput, cedarwood, clary sage, cypress, frankincense, geranium, juniper, lavender, lemon, lemongrass, lime, mandarin, palmarosa, peppermint, rosewood, sandalwood, tea tree, ylang ylang

perspiration Cypress, lemongrass, tea tree

psoriasis Benzoin, bergamot, chamomile, lavender, tea tree, yarrow

rejuvenate Carrot seed, frankincense, lavender, myrrh, neroli, rosewood

scabies Lemon, lemongrass, peppermint, rosemary, thyme

scars Carrot seed, jasmine, mandarin, neroli, patchouli

sensitive Chamomile, geranium, jasmine, neroli, lavender, rose

sunburn Clary sage, lavender, peppermint

ulcers Frankincense, geranium, juniper, lavender, myrrh, tea tree

varicose veins Cypress, geranium, ginger, lemon, neroli, tea tree, yarrow

warts and verrucae Lemon, lime, tea tree

wounds and sores Benzoin, frankincense, geranium, juniper, myrrh, patchouli, tea tree, thyme

wrinkles Carrot seed, clary sage, frankincense, myrrh, palmarosa, patchouli, rose, rosemary, rosewood

Supplies

Denise Brown Essential Oils
MWB Business Exchange
23 Hinton Road
Bournemouth BH1 2EF
Tel: +44 (0)1202 708887
www.denisebrown.co.uk

A wide selection of high quality pure unadulterated essential oils, base oils, creams and lotions, relaxation music, etc. is available from Denise Brown Essential Oils (International Mail Order)

Aromatherapy Training and Therapists

Beaumont College of Natural Medicine
MWB Business Exchange
Hinton Road
Bournemouth BH1 2EF
Tel: +44 (0)1202 708887
www.beaumontcollege.co.uk

Information on training courses under the direction of Denise Brown

International Federation of Professional Aromatherapists
82 Ashby Road
Hinckley
Leics. LE10 1SN
Tel: +44 (0)1455 637987
www.ifparoma.org

Send s.a.e for a list of qualified therapists in your area

Aromatherapy Organisations Council
The AOC Secretary
PO Box 19834
London SE25 6WF
Tel : +44 (0)208 251 7912 Fax : +44 (0)208 251 7942
www.aocuk.net

Aromatherapy On-Line Correspondence Course
www.beaumontcollege.co.uk/correspond.html

Correspondence/interactive internet aromatherapy e-course for use on friends and family

Overseas

American Alliance of Aromatherapy
P.O. Box 750428
Petaluma
CA 94975-0428
USA

American Botanical Council
P.O. Box 201660
Austin
TX 78720-1660
USA

National Association of Holistic Aromatherapy
P.O. Box 17622
Boulder
CO 80308
USA

Further Reading

To complement the information in this book why not read Denise Brown's other books in this series:
Teach Yourself Massage (Hodder & Stoughton)
Teach Yourself Hand Reflexology (Hodder & Stoughton)
Teach Yourself Indian Head Massage (Hodder & Stoughton)
Available from most literary outlets.

index

teach® yourself

Afrikaans
Access 2002
Accounting, Basic
Alexander Technique
Algebra
Arabic
Arabic Script, Beginner's
Aromatherapy
Astronomy
Bach Flower Remedies
Bengali
Better Chess
Better Handwriting
Biology
Body Language
Book Keeping
Book Keeping & Accounting
Brazilian Portuguese
Bridge
Buddhism
Buddhism, 101 Key Ideas
Bulgarian
Business Studies
Business Studies, 101 Key Ideas
C++
Calculus
Calligraphy
Cantonese
Card Games
Catalan
Chemistry, 101 Key Ideas
Chess
Chi Kung
Chinese
Chinese, Beginner's

Chinese Language, Life & Culture
Chinese Script, Beginner's
Christianity
Classical Music
Copywriting
Counselling
Creative Writing
Crime Fiction
Croatian
Crystal Healing
Czech
Danish
Desktop Publishing
Digital Photography
Digital Video & PC Editing
Drawing
Dream Interpretation
Dutch
Dutch, Beginner's
Dutch Dictionary
Dutch Grammar
Eastern Philosophy
ECDL
E-Commerce
Economics, 101 Key Ideas
Electronics
English, American (EFL)
English as a Foreign Language
English, Correct
English Grammar
English Grammar (EFL)
English, Instant, for French Speakers
English, Instant, for German Speakers
English, Instant, for Italian Speakers
English, Instant, for Spanish Speakers

English for International Business
English Language, Life & Culture
English Verbs
English Vocabulary
Ethics
Excel 2002
Feng Shui
Film Making
Film Studies
Finance for non-Financial Managers
Finnish
Flexible Working
Flower Arranging
French
French, Beginner's
French Grammar
French Grammar, Quick Fix
French, Instant
French, Improve your
French Language, Life & Culture
French Starter Kit
French Verbs
French Vocabulary
Gaelic
Gaelic Dictionary
Gardening
Genetics
Geology
German
German, Beginner's
German Grammar
German Grammar, Quick Fix
German, Instant
German, Improve your
German Language, Life & Culture
German Verbs
German Vocabulary
Go
Golf
Greek
Greek, Ancient
Greek, Beginner's
Greek, Instant
Greek, New Testament
Greek Script, Beginner's
Guitar
Gulf Arabic
Hand Reflexology
Hebrew, Biblical
Herbal Medicine
Hieroglyphics
Hindi
Hindi, Beginner's
Hindi Script, Beginner's

teach
yourself

massage
denise whichello brown

- Do you want to understand the principles of massage?
- Would you like your life to benefit from this popular technique?
- Do you need a simple introduction in preparation for a course of study?

Massage gives a complete guide to this ancient and popular technique. Learn how to apply the basic principles to relieve stress, to treat sports injuries or to develop your personal relationships. The text is extensively illustrated with clear, fully labelled diagrams.

Denise Whichello Brown is a highly acclaimed practitioner, lecturer and author of international repute, with over 20 years' experience in complementary medicine.

teach
yourself

indian head massage
denise whichello brown

- Do you want to know more about this ancient therapy?
- Do you want to understand the basic principles?
- Are you looking for a therapy you can apply to your own life?

Indian Head Massage is a comprehensive introduction to this ancient holistic therapy that balances body, mind and spirit to promote health and well-being. The book explains the origins and benefits of Indian head massage and its basic techniques, and gives clear, step-by-step instructions. Use the simple treatments to improve the health and well-being of yourself and others.

Denise Whichello Brown is a highly acclaimed practitioner, lecturer and author of international repute, with over 20 years' experience in complementary medicine.

teach
yourself

hand reflexology
denise whichello brown

- Do you want to discover an ideal way of treating yourself?
- Are you looking for an easy-to-follow guide to basic hand reflexology techniques?
- Do you want to know how to treat and eliminate many common medical problems?

Hand Reflexology is a simple, straightforward and practical guide to this ancient and increasingly popular healing art. Discover how reflexology has an enormous part to play in healthcare and how it offers much more than just a hand massage. Explore the roots of reflexology, and learn techniques easily with step-by-step instructions with accompanying illustrations.

Denise Whichello Brown is internationally recognized as an accomplished practioner and lecturer in the field of complemetary medicine.

teach yourself

reflexology
chris stormer

- Are you new to reflexology?
- Would you like to learn a different approach to good health?
- Do you want to relieve stress?

Reflexology will help you to discover this ancient and gentle form of healing, which uses reflex points on the feet to stimulate the body's natural ability to heel itself. The step-by-step instructions and many illustrations give even the complete beginner the information and confidence to get started right away.

Chris Stormer is an acknowledged authority on reflexology. She is the founder of the Reflexology Academy of Southern Africa and holds workshops and lectures worldwide.